The *Healing Touch of* Massage

The Healing Touch of Massage

Carlo de Paoli

Photography by Sue Atkinson

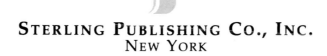

STERLING PUBLISHING CO., INC.
NEW YORK

I would like to dedicate this book to all the bodyworkers past and present who use and have used body therapy to treat the whole being.

Library of Congress Cataloging-in-Publication Data Available

2 4 6 8 10 9 7 5 3 1

Published 1995 by Sterling Publishing Company, Inc.
387 Park Avenue South, New York, N.Y. 10016

Originally published in Great Britain by
Headline Book Publishing, a division of Hodder Headline PLC
338 Euston Road, London NW1 3BH
under the title *Massage and Bodywork for Health*
Text copyright © 1995 by Carlo De Paoli
Photographs copyright © 1995 by Sue Atkinson
This edition copyright © 1995 by Eddison Sadd Editions
Distributed in Canada by Sterling Publishing
c/o Canadian Manda Group, One Atlantic Avenue, Suite 105
Toronto, Ontario, Canada M6K 3E7

AN EDDISON · SADD EDITION
Edited, designed and produced by
Eddison Sadd Editions Limited
St Chad's Court
146B King's Cross Road
London WC1X 9DH

Phototypeset in Meridien and Americana Bold by
SX Composing Ltd, Rayleigh, UK
Origination by Tipongraph Srl, Italy
Produced by Mandarin Offset, printed and bound in Hong Kong

Sterling ISBN 0-8069-1359-2

Contents

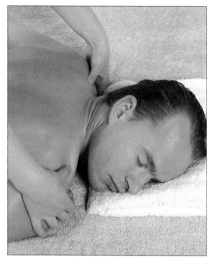

Thumb Pressure

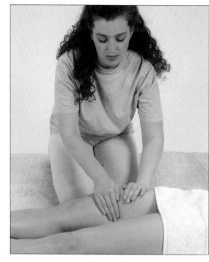

Wringing

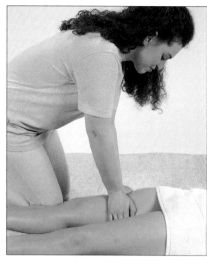

Palm Pressure

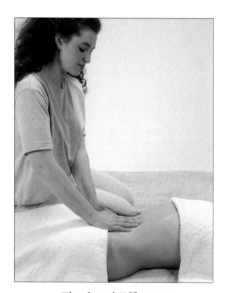

Flat-hand Effleurage

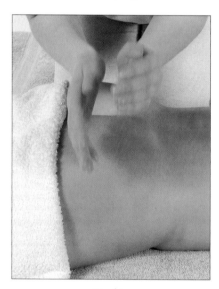

Hacking

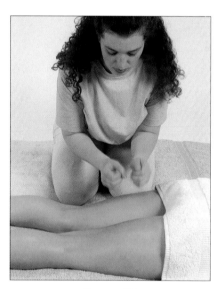

Pummelling

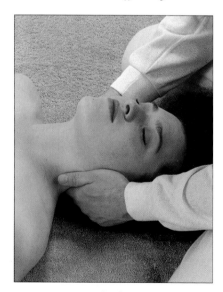

Articulation

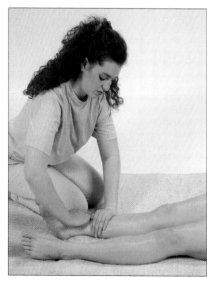

Cupped-hand Effleurage

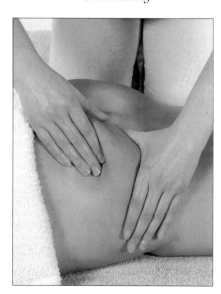

Kneading

PART ONE
Massage Techniques

Part One sets the scene for a life-time of health-giving massage aided by the use of aromatherapy and herbalism. The history of the art of massage over the centuries, from ancient Indian massage to the more contemporary Swedish approach, is all here. And the benefits of massage, to soothe and allay many common complaints as well as maintain a healthy body to resist ailments, are outlined.

The principles of each school of therapy – Swedish and Eastern massage, shiatsu, osteopathy, neuro-muscular massage, aromatherapy and herbalism – are all set out. Then the types of touch – from effleurage to acupressure and percussion to articulation – that you will use in the massage sequences in Part Two are clearly explained.

Finally, there is a section on how to prepare yourself for a massage treatment, both mentally and physically, preparing the treatment room and the massage receiver. Now you are ready to begin your massage.

With a firm grasp of the principles and techniques laid out here you can feel confident to move on to Part Two where you will learn how to put them into practice.

The History and Benefits of Massage

Recent research suggests that massage, as a form of therapy, was already in use several centuries before the birth of Christ. Mentioned in ancient Greek, Egyptian, Indian and Chinese medical texts, it played a particularly important role in the traditional medicine of the Far East and India and, throughout history, was taught along with other therapies, such as herbalism, exercise and acupuncture. Homer, who lived around the eighth century BC, mentioned it in his book, *Odyssey*, as a restorative treatment for warriors; about the fourth century BC, Hippocrates, the father of Western medicine, made extensive use of it for the treatment and prevention of diseases; and so did the renowned physician Galen (AD 150) who is recognized as the major authority of traditional Western herbalism. In ancient Egypt, massage was taught in temples as a sacred art alongside herbal medicine and other forms of religious rituals and divination.

The Art of Massage

Massage has been used also, throughout history, as a form of relaxation and beauty treatment. It was particularly popular with the ancient Romans. Base oils were mixed with essential oils and herbs, and applied with full-body massage techniques to regenerate and beautify the skin, especially the skin of the face. The ointments were attributed with various properties, some factual, some vastly exaggerated. Certainly it must have been a real treat to spend all day at the Roman Baths indulging oneself with hot vapours, swimming and then being massaged with aromatic ointments!

Unfortunately, after the fall of the Roman empire, the Western world adopted a more puritanical view of life, and any so-called pampering of the body was viewed as sinful. As a result, massage, both as a form of relaxation and as a form of medicine, was ostracized. This situation remained for several centuries, and in Europe it was not until the end of the eighteenth century that the relaxing and therapeutic effects of massage witnessed a true revival.

The art of massage is as ancient as touch itself. Both human beings and animals have always been endowed with the intuitive knowledge that stroking and caressing with a caring, loving attitude brings comfort, relaxation and general well-being. In our scientifically-minded age, studies have overwhelmingly confirmed that a loving touch can also relieve pain, soothe sorrows, promote health, and ensure the growth and development of happy healthy offspring, both human and animal. Studies of children and young animals, such as monkeys, have confirmed this fact time and time again.

As far as plants are concerned, the book, *Secret Life of Plants*, by Tompkins and Bird, has sold over a million copies and dramatically changed people's perception of other forms of life. It certainly had a remarkable impact on me. In their book, Tompkins and Bird cite many experiments that show that even plants are endowed with intelligence and feelings, and have a tremendous response to touch, words and, perhaps even more astonishingly, to thoughts. For example, plants that are regularly touched and sent loving thoughts are now known to grow far more strongly than plants that are deprived of such contact.

The essence of massage, then, is a loving,

caring touch – whether it is applied in a family, between friends or in a therapeutic situation – which throughout the ages has become structured into healing techniques.

In this book, I use the word 'bodywork' to indicate advanced forms of massage, such as shiatsu or osteopathy, where therapeutic treatments on the musculoskeletal system – the body's main framework of bones, joints, muscles and ligaments – aim to correct particular imbalances by using various manipulative methods such as stretching or rocking the joints. I give you an overview of the advantages and applications of massage and bodywork, and outline all the possibilities as each body system is examined in detail.

Massage brings people together. Where there is conflict and misunderstanding, it calms tensions and creates unity by engendering feelings of closeness and tenderness. The following story illustrates this point.

Creating Love and Harmony

In ancient Japan a recently-married young woman had, according to custom, moved into her husband's home where his parents also resided. After a while she visited a Buddhist monk, and, with tears in her eyes, expressed her frustration with her mother-in-law who was constantly bullying her. She was so desperate that she asked the monk to teach her a way by which she could gradually kill her mother-in-law without arousing any suspicion. The monk replied that he knew the perfect way for her to achieve her aim, and set about teaching her a form of massage through which she could gradually kill the old woman.

A few weeks later the same young woman returned to the monk in a state of great agitation. The monk enquired whether his method was working, and the woman immediately begged him to show her how to undo the harm that she might have done.

The monk feigned surprise and asked what had brought about this change of heart and mind. She answered that, after a few weeks of

regularly massaging her mother-in-law in the way that he had taught her, she had grown very fond of her and now they both loved each other very much. The monk then smilingly explained that it had never been his intention to show her a way to hurt anybody, quite the contrary. He had taught her massage to bring them both together, thus creating love and harmony in her family life.

How Massage Helps the Main Body Systems

The nervous system operates rather like a vast electrical network which, along with the endocrine system, interconnects and harmonizes all the individual parts of the body. The nervous system, for example, monitors our blood pressure, rate of breathing, digestive phases, and relates this information to the brain which, in turn, transmits signals through nerve pathways to keep the body in balance. It also regulates the relationship with the external environment by relating information to the brain through the five senses – hearing, sight, taste, touch and smell – and then receiving instructions on how to act.

The nervous system is greatly affected by stress and can, as a result, either become hyperactive (frenetic) or hypoactive (underactive). In the first condition, to use Eastern phraseology, we can be said to have an excess of Yang (active principle of nature) and in the second, excess of Yin (passive principle of nature). These disharmonies of two natural and essential forces can, in turn, unbalance many of our physiological activities and contribute to or create various conditions such as headaches and indigestion.

Massage and bodywork, with their great variety of healing strokes, can be very effective in balancing the nervous system and restoring homeostasis (physical balance and equilibrium). The skin and muscles contain many nerve endings and connections, and the soothing, balancing, healing touch of massage is relayed by them to every part of the body to bring relief and promote well-being.

By contracting and extending, the skeletal muscles create movements in various parts of the body. They can, however, become painful and contracted with spasms and abnormal tissue, as seen for example in fibrositis, and they can store toxins such as lactic acid. In certain conditions they can waste, becoming weak and flaccid. Such conditions can make some movements difficult, painful or even impossible.

Massage can stretch and regenerate the muscles restoring normal elasticity (suppleness) and strength (stamina). Sports people, for example, greatly benefit from massage treatment. So can everyone else – the young to grow up with healthy muscles and the old to avoid flabbiness, muscle wastage and weakness.

Freeing the Body

All bone movements occur at joints, as in the shoulder, neck, knee, hip, spine, and so on. Many schools of healing, such as yoga in the East and osteopathy in the West, believe that long-lasting youth and good health depend a great deal upon the flexibility of joints. Bodywork concentrates on releasing the joints and thus contributes to keeping the body upright, agile and as free as possible from arthritic conditions.

Most nerves, veins and arteries pass through the joints and muscles and, as a result, abnormalities and restrictions within the muscular and skeletal systems can greatly hamper the healthy functioning of a body's metabolism. For example the vagus nerve, which originates in the skull, passes into the neck from an area located at the base of the skull and the first cervical or neck vertebra. Muscular and joint restrictions around this area can impinge upon the vagus nerve, which contributes to the regulation of a wide range of organs and functions, such as the pharynx and most thoracic and abdominal organs. When obstructed it disrupts some of the functions involved in breathing and respiration. This example illustrates how massage work on the neck can improve respiration and digestion.

The sciatic nerve originates from the lumbar and sacral area in the lower back, passes through the buttocks and descends into the leg and foot. This nerve can be impinged by muscles and joints in the lower back and often by a contraction of buttock muscles. This, in turn, can lead to pain in the lower leg and occasionally in the foot. Therefore, we can see how by mobilizing and massaging the lower part of the trunk we can resolve pain in the leg.

Nerves originating from the sacrum control organs in the lower abdomen, such as the descending colon, kidneys, bladder and reproductive organs. By working around the sacro-iliac joints and lumbar area all these organs can be revitalized. I once had a patient who became impotent after receiving a powerful karate kick in the lower back that slightly displaced his sacrum. By gently mobilizing his lower back, his sexual functions were fully restored.

Improving Circulation

Massage also exerts a beneficial pumping action on the circulatory system by gently squeezing and releasing the muscles and circulatory vessels that pass through it. This improves blood circulation by favouring the exchange, at a cellular level, of fresh nutrient-full blood, to blood that is carrying toxins away from the cells.

It works in the same way on the lymphatic system by favouring the passage of lymph (fluid carrying nutrients and white blood cells to body tissues, and waste matter away from them) into the bloodstream and thus promoting detoxification. In this way, massage exerts an important influence on the regenerative and cleansing capabilities of the body.

This book shows you how, in a simple, concise, step-by-step way, to use the various massage and bodywork techniques to improve all the functions of the body while, at the same time, relaxing and revitalizing the mind. It also shows you how to enhance the massage techniques by giving practical advice on essential oils, herbs, diet and exercise.

Schools of Therapy

Since the dramatic improvements in international communication and travel, we have all become increasingly attracted to each other's cultures. This interest has encompassed most spheres of human life. At first it seemed that it was mainly the West exporting its ways abroad and from the 1920s onwards, the whole world seemed to adopt the Western medical system and ways of life. In recent years, however, there has been a dramatic change.

The West has discovered aspects of foreign culture, particularly Eastern, that have greatly improved its quality of life, physically, emotionally, mentally and spiritually. Acupuncture, shiatsu, Chinese herbal medicine, yoga, and many other healing traditions, are now part of our awareness and way of life, and we have all benefited from this integrated vision.

When this realization is applied to massage and bodywork, it contributes a great deal to broadening and improving the scope and efficiency of manual therapy. For example, in general terms, Western forms of bodywork are good for working with the body in an anatomical and muscular way, while Eastern forms of bodywork are good for working at a more vital energetic level. If they complement each other, they improve health and well-being.

This book aims to assist this healing process and show how various approaches, which complement each other, can be harmoniously blended. Accompanied by advice on essential oils, herbs, diet and exercise, I am confident that *Massage and Bodywork for Health* will become and remain a good companion for life.

Swedish Massage

Per Henrik Ling of Sweden (1776-1839) is acclaimed in the West as the father of modern massage. He was a devoted and enthusiastic massage therapist who dedicated his life to the development and acceptance of this healing art throughout Europe. He realized that it was advisable for the person giving the massage to have a certain knowledge of anatomy and physiology.

With this aim he created training centres which taught Swedish massage and exercise. He introduced, among others, such terms as effleurage (gentle rhythmic stroking) which is used everywhere on the body to improve circulation and petrissage (kneading, wringing and rubbing), which is used to squeeze toxins and tensions out of muscles.

His method, which is based on various ancient traditional massage practices, combines therapeutic massage with exercises for muscles and joints. It was largely due to his penchant for using a base oil when massaging that the use of various oils with their life-enhancing qualities became increasingly popular in

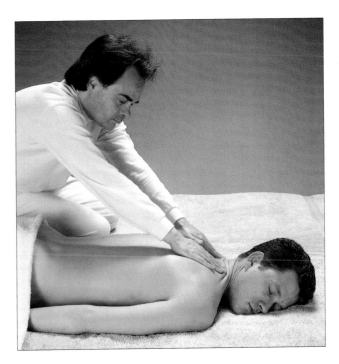

Effleurage, which means 'stroking', is a gentle rhythmical massage stroke that is used all over the body. It relaxes muscles for deeper pressure massage work, eases tensions and pain, and improves circulation of blood and lymph. It also relaxes the whole person.

To stimulate a healing flow of energy along the body's meridians (energy paths) shiatsu uses, for example, thumb, finger, palm, heel of hand pressure, and stretching techniques.

With the same aim in mind, acupressure uses firm thumb or fingertip pressure along a system of pain-relieving pressure points, called acupoints, which lie on the meridian.

The aim of these techniques is to stimulate the meridian along which energy flows.

Shown right is a shiatsu stretching technique applied to the pelvis to alleviate tension and pain, and restore freedom of movement.

Shown below is a thumb pressure being applied to Pericardium 6 (PE 6) (pericardium are membranes which surround the heart). Pressure is applied here to release anxiety and tension, to soothe pain and cramp, and to promote good circulation.

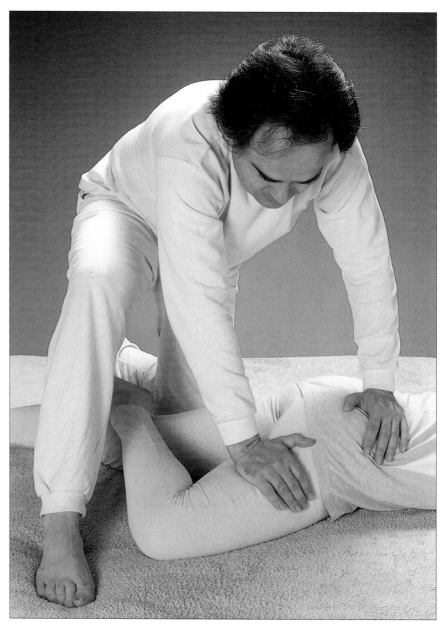

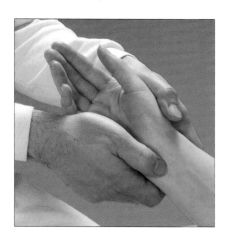

Europe in the nineteenth century and are still used for all forms of massage today.

The main aim, then, of Swedish massage is to improve circulation, manipulate joints, and stretch and release muscles throughout the body to create a variety of beneficial effects.

Eastern Massage

In order to explain the Eastern forms of massage, such as acupressure and shiatsu, I will give a brief introduction to the basic concepts of Chinese medicine for those who are not familiar with them. First, in the East medicine is part of an all-encompassing philosophical and religious vision of life. The universe is viewed as a unity where opposites complement each other and always seek a level of harmony. Disease occurs when this harmony is broken. Western thought, however, has had a tendency to separate the material and spiritual levels.

Qi, the subtle and vital force of energy, so often referred to in oriental therapy, runs through the body in meridians – clearly defined channels – each of which is connected to and influences a major organ of the body. When the vital Qi force flows freely there is health and well-being; when the flow of Qi is disrupted there is a blockage leading to problems.

The meridians are best visualized as flowing rivers where, at certain key points, the current and power of the river is stronger and even visible from the surface. These points along the meridians of the human body are known as the acupoints. Through these points – used in acupressure, acupuncture and shiatsu – the energy can be contacted to maintain or to restore a life-and-health enhancing flow. Massage, using these points, is included in each chapter.

Osteopathy

This system of physical manipulation of joints and bodywork, which originated in America around 1870, was created by Dr Andrew Still (1828–1917). Although osteopathy has only recently become a widely-practised mainstream medical system, its principles have been practised for centuries.

Dr Still noticed that health problems arise when part of the body's main-frame structure of bones, joints, muscles and ligaments gets out of alignment, and that manipulation can bring about release, restore mobility, eliminate congestion and dramatically improve health-related problems. For example, when a joint is impeded and/or deviates from the norm, arteries and nerves can become pinched and obstructed, and give rise to trouble. Freeing the joints through manual manipulation results in better circulation and enables the various body structures and organs that were formerly starved of fresh blood to regenerate themselves and thrive again. Muscle agility and lymphatic drainage can also be improved in this way.

Chiropractors are somewhat similar to osteopaths. They treat a range of disorders through the manipulation of joints, muscles and, especially, the spine. Chiropractors make much greater use of X-rays and conventional diagnostic techniques than do osteopaths.

Osteopathy is, of course, best known as an effective system for treating problems of the

Necks are notorious for accumulating tensions, which result in stiffness and painful limited movement. The neck-stretching techniques, used by osteopaths, are a very effective way to articulate and maintain the natural movements of the neck, and to restore freedom of movement when health problems occur. The restoration may take time and patience, but the dispelling of muscular spasms and pain means the time is well spent.

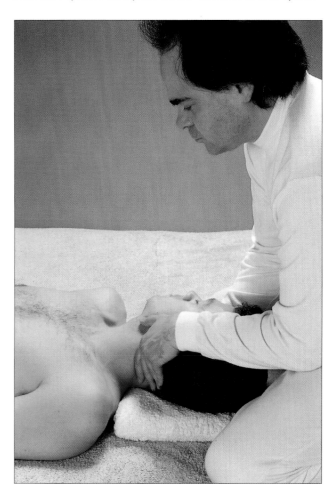

musculoskeletal structure, such as back pain, and many modern osteopaths concentrate their energies on manipulating and freeing spinal-column restrictions.

Dr Still concentrated on safe ways to stretch and mobilize the musculoskeletal system. Later on, many of his followers turned towards high velocity techniques (what people know as 'cracks' or express as 'I am going to the osteopath to have my back cracked'). These particular techniques can be very effective in freeing joint restrictions, but, in my opinion, there is no substitute for a more integrated

Neuro-muscular massage uses friction techniques applied mainly with the thumbs to release muscular contractions and tension. Use for most muscular areas of the body.

Here it is being applied to free rib restrictions where massaging the intercostal muscles increases respiratory capability and lung function. The masseur is using his left arm to stretch the rib cage, and the thumb of his right hand to massage the intercostal muscles in the space between the ribs. This technique frees spasms in the rib muscles benefitting the respiratory system.

Neuro-muscular massage has inspired other bodywork techniques, such as Rolfing, which aims to align the body by massaging connective tissue and muscles; it is practised still by osteopaths.

Applied to the back it increases flexibility and prevents problems like fibrositis. Used on the legs it improves circulation by freeing muscular constrictions in the veins and arteries.

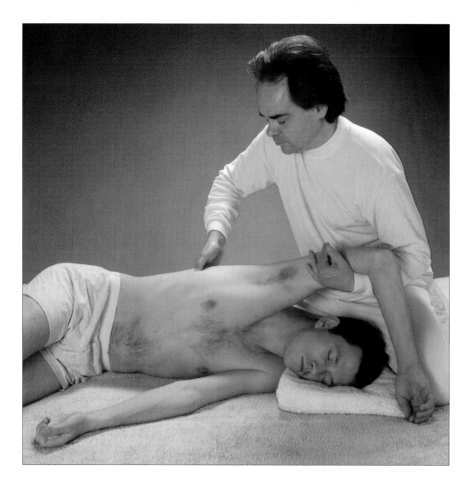

bodywork approach that includes using the hands to massage, stretch and manipulate the framework of bones, joints, muscles and ligaments to counteract problems and restore normal function. Fortunately, many of the early osteopathic techniques, based on massage methods, are now safely incorporated into bodywork systems.

Neuro-muscular Massage

This approach to bodywork was developed by Stanley Lief, a chiropractor and naturopath, born in the 1890s. In the 1920s–30s, his approach in treating illnesses with bodywork techniques and nature cures gained a large following, particularly in England.

Neuro-muscular massage concentrates on releasing muscular contraction and tension that can create conditions such as fibrositis. These muscular abnormalities can restrict movement of joints and disrupt many bodily functions.

Neuro-muscular techniques tend to use friction and pressure techniques applied especially with the thumbs. This can be applied to most muscular areas of the body, and I frequently use it to free rib restrictions. Working, for example, on the intercostal muscles increases respiratory capability and improves lung function. If the lungs are restricted they cannot expand properly to fill with the cleansing and revitalizing oxygen that is so essential to the health of the body, and they are also unable to eliminate carbon dioxide fully.

Aromatherapy

Many plants, flowers and wood resins contain glands filled with a volatile aromatic oil that is called an essential oil. By volatile we mean an oil that quickly evaporates on contact with air in contrast to a fatty oil that sinks in and remains in the place that it penetrates. For example, if you rub a leaf containing essential

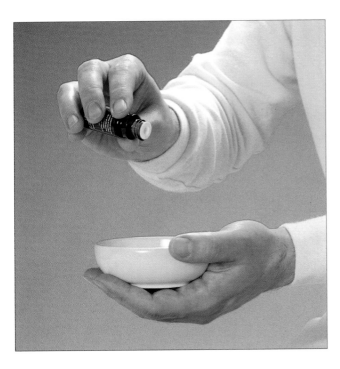

Most essential oils, which are added to a base oil (see above) for massage, have anti-bacterial qualities that preserve skin tissue and block the spread of infection. Some, such as lavender, also have an analgesic action so are useful for reducing pain. Essential oils are extracted from plants by steam distillation.

POINTS TO NOTE

• Some people are allergic to certain essential oils, so always try a tiny amount to test the skin's reaction. This applies to essential oils added to bath water as well as those used in massage.
• Do not use essential oils when pregnant, when breast-feeding, or for massaging babies or children under twelve, except under the guidance of a qualified aromatherapist.
• Oils should never be taken internally except under medical supervision.
• Essential oils deteriorate and evaporate rapidly when exposed to heat, sunlight or damp. Store in dark glass bottles or metal containers with airtight lids or stoppers, and keep them in a cool, dark, dry place.
• Once diluted in a base oil, essential oils will last for two-to-three months, if correctly stored in a refrigerator.
• When beginning a massage, pour the diluted oil into the palm of your hand, rub your hands together gently to warm it and then oil the body before you begin to massage.

oil against your hand, the fragrance of its essence will evaporate after a little while; if, however, you put a drop of olive oil on a tissue the stain soaks in and remains.

The essential oil in a plant gives it a unique fragrance or 'personality'. Research into understanding the function of these volatile oils is still underway, but one of their main purposes is defensive. With their many highly-antiseptic properties they repel harmful germs and insects which would endanger the survival of the plant. Laboratory experiments have shown how essential oils kill bacteria making them useful in skin infections, grazes and cuts. They have also been used throughout the ages in creams and perfumes.

As you read on, you will find advice on how to use essential oils to complement and enhance the various massage techniques.

Preparing Oils for Massage

Essential oils need to be diluted with a base oil, sometimes called 'carrier oils' (for example, almond, grapeseed, unrefined vegetable, extra virgin olive, sunflower seed oil). For a full-body massage, prepare a saucer containing 30 ml (2 tablespoons) of your chosen base massage oil and add three drops of your preferred essential oils. If you are using only one essential oil, then use three drops; if you are using three different essential oils, then use one drop of each.

The Properties of Essential Oils

Essential oils are mentioned as healing accompaniments to massage throughout this book. The following is a brief description of their healing properties, and what they are used for. The advice for people who are not experts in aromatherapy is to keep to the recommended dosages and only to use the oils externally.

Aniseed *(Pimpinella anisum)*
This oil acts as a sedative on the nervous system. It helps digestion, relieving flatulence and nervous indigestion; calms coughing spasms,

and helps expectoration. To alleviate colic, rub on the stomach of a small child, but do not use more than one drop to 30 ml (2 tablespoons) of base oil; adults double this amount, but do not repeat it more than twice a week in either case because of its sedative properties.

Benzoin *(Styrax benzoin)*

This improves the respiratory system by aiding expectoration, while calming coughing spasms. With both an expectorant and soothing action, it is useful for colds, flu and sore throats.

Bergamot *(Citrus bergamia)*

Medical research shows that past use, diluted as a douche to treat urinary and vaginal infections, may have led to problems of the female reproductive system. Has a beneficial effect on the nervous system and an anti-depressant action, its pleasant scent lifts the spirits.

Chamomile *(Chamaemelum nobile syn. Anthemis nobile)*

This oil has a marked effect on the nervous and digestive systems, particularly when indigestion is due to stress and worry; for this, massage the abdomen. It is a good remedy for pain and a useful anti-inflammatory agent; good for skin irritations characterized by redness. Recommended for restlessness and insomnia.

Clary sage *(Salvia sclarea)*

Used in preference to common sage because, while sharing many of its properties, it is far less toxic. It has a pronounced action on the respiratory and nervous systems, and is used for people who have a weak chest, tire easily and suffer from shortness of breath. People who lack will-power and self-confidence find it gives energy and lifts depression.

Cypress *(Cupressus sempervirens)*

This is mainly used to improve the functioning of the circulatory system. It exerts a stimulating and astringent action. It strengthens the valves of the veins, helping conditions such as varicose veins, and promotes the flow of blood through-out the body. Do not massage varicose veins; apply the oil to areas such as the feet and hands.

Eucalyptus *(Eucalyptus globulus)*

This is recommended universally for respiratory problems and infections. It is used mostly for colds and flu where mucus is present. The expectorant action makes it useful for chesty and catarrhal conditions like bronchitis, when it is used as an inhalant (dissolve about ten drops in very hot water and breathe the vapour).

Fennel *(Foeniculum vulgare)*

Primarily used for improving digestion, it alleviates flatulence, abdominal swelling and discomfort; also intestinal conditions such as constipation and irritable bowel syndrome. With a mild expectorant action, it can be used for catarrh. Considered a good diuretic.

Frankincense *(Boswellia thurifera)*

Reputed to lift the spirits, calm the mind and dispel depression. It also acts on the respiratory system by calming a cough and expelling mucus. It improves circulation; and tones up the skin. When massaged with lavender on an injured area it can hasten recovery and soothe the pain.

Geranium *(Pelargonium odoratissimum)*

This is balancing, soothing, gently calming; it does not sedate and tones without exciting. Promotes relaxation, leaving you alert and fresh; is an excellent anti-inflammatory oil, helping skin conditions characterized by redness and dryness; mildly astringent, it helps varicose veins; massaged over the abdomen, reduces diarrhoea.

Ginger *(Zingiber officinale)*

Warming for body and mind, this is recommended for people who suffer from cold symptoms. Treats poor circulation, colds and flu, and alleviates fatigue; is a particularly good expectorant, used for coughs and bronchitis. Also stimulates digestion, reduces nausea. Popular travel sickness remedy in tea or capsule form.

Jasmine *(Jasminum officinale, J. grandiflorum)*
This enlivens the heart, opens the chest and lifts depression. Unlike some 'hot' essential oils, it increases vitality without overheating the system, and, at the same time, encourages joy and enthusiasm. I feel it is the best and safest aphrodisiac for massaging the lower back area.

Juniper *(Juniperus communis)*
The stimulating properties of this oil are recommended for general debility. Not recommended for acute inflammation of the kidneys, but is a diuretic. Useful for rheumatism, particularly when worsened by cold and damp weather.

Lavender *(Lavandula vera, L. officinalis)*
This is probably one of the most popular, potent, multi-use essential oils. It regulates the central nervous system, acting as a useful sedative for anxiety, insomnia and hysteria. It calms pain and is used for complaints such as neuritis and nerve pain such as sciatica. It is a disinfectant and helps to heal cuts, bruises and abrasions, skin irritations, chilblains and bee stings. It improves circulation and muscular cramps. Because of its potent sedative qualities, it should not be used as a body massage more than twice a week.

Lemon balm *(Melissa officinalis)*
This oil can cause skin irritation and should be used only in small amounts. It is good for stress and tension, headaches, nervous indigestion, sadness, depression and nervous exhaustion.

Mandarin peel *(Citrus × nobilis)*
This oil decongests the liver, and is useful for pain and discomfort in the right flank accompanied by a bitter taste in the mouth. It helps digestion, alleviating flatulence and belching, and has a mild astringent quality helpful in diarrhoea. It is also used as an expectorant.

Marjoram *(Origanum majorana)*
Marjoram is highly regarded for its action on the respiratory system and on the nervous system. Very few plants have such a complementary action as marjoram when there is the need to combine tonic and calming actions. For example, there are individuals who are highly stressed and tense yet at the same time feel tired and fatigued. Marjoram can solve this problem by increasing stamina while calming tension. It also soothes coughing spasms, strengthens the lungs and promotes expectoration; and is used for treating muscular aches and pains and arthritis.

Neroli *(Citrus aurantium)*
One of the best calming and relaxing oils without sedating or creating drowsiness; it is recommended for insomnia, anxiety and stress.

Orange peel *(Citrus sinensis)*
This helps to regulate liver functioning, soothing right flank pain and the bitter taste in the mouth. Good for digestion, especially when abdominal discomfort is accompanied by constipation, where it blends well with essential oil of fennel. Has a calming effect without being a sedative.

Peppermint *(Mentha piperita)*
Acts primarily on the digestive system, stimulating the digestive processes. Alleviates flatulence, belching and abdominal swelling; has a stimulating, refreshing effect on the whole body. Widely used for colds and flu and assists expectoration.

Rose *(Rosa × damascena, R. gallica)*
These oils relax, create trust and open the heart to love. They help irregular and painful menstruation. They contain anti-inflammatory and slightly astringent properties, making them useful for skin problems. They cleanse the liver and help the digestive system. They alleviate anxiety and encourage relaxation and cheerfulness.

Rosemary *(Rosmarinus officinalis)*
This stimulating, warming oil improves poor circulation and a weak blood flow to the brain resulting in symptoms such as poor memory and concentration. Stimulates the liver and increases appetite; used to treat people who suffer from cold and lethargy, and arthritis

made worse by cold weather. Avoid in cases of high blood pressure and all complaints accompanied by hot sensations and inflammation.

Sandalwood *(Santalum album)*

This oil promotes peace of mind, meditation and spiritual thoughts. It encourages clear thinking in difficult situations. With its anti-inflammatory and soothing nature, it is used for urinary infections and diarrhoea.

Tea-tree *(Melaleuca alternifolia)*

This is renowned for its effective action against bacteria, fungi and viruses. Massage over the bladder area for thrush infections or cystitis. Use in the bath to help various skin problems, particularly if fungal. A drop added to water as a face wash can improve acne.

Thyme *(Thymus vulgaris)*

Thyme yields a very strong, hot and pungent essential oil which should be used only in very small amounts. One drop added to a bath or to 30 ml (2 tablespoons) of massage oil is more than enough. Thyme has a very powerful action on the respiratory system; eliminates harmful germs; is a very effective expectorant; and is good for bronchitis. It has a toning stimulating action; avoid in cases of high blood pressure.

Vetiver *(Vetiveria zizanoides)*

Produces a pleasant sense of languor and relaxation, while refreshing the mind. Very good for the circulation; for treating hot inflamed extremities, and inflamed dry skin conditions.

Ylang-ylang *(Cananga odorata)*

This oil promotes serenity and joy. It has a sweet scent and is highly popular as a relaxant and aphrodisiac; prescribed for sexual inadequacy when caused by anxiety and apprehension.

Herbal Medicine

Herbal medicine, which can be regarded as an extension of nutrition, is one of the pillars of natural healing, and I have included through-out this book herbal recipes accompanied by advice for each body system. The recipes are simple, safe to use, and based on herbs and spices that are widely available.

The therapeutic use of herbs is as old as mankind itself, for even animals instinctively search for herbs, grasses and leaves to treat themselves. The first humans had the same intuitive contact with nature and, over thousands of years, the use of herbs has evolved into a worldwide healing system.

As one of the most ancient systems of natural treatment, herbal medicine has the advantage of having been enriched by the experience of countless practitioners – and, to name but a few countries, the ancient civilizations of Egypt, Greece, Rome, India and China, relied on a sophisticated system of plant healing. This ancient knowledge has been – and is still being – enriched by present-day scientific research. Today's pharmaceutical companies are searching constantly for new compounds that can be extracted from plants, and many existing medical prescriptions are plant-based.

Using Herbal Preparations

There are many ways in which herbal preparations can be administered, but in this book I have concentrated on two main ones.

Infusions. Thoroughly mix the chosen herbal mixture, and then infuse 5 mg (1 teaspoon) in a cup of hot water. Cover and let it stand for five-to-ten minutes. Strain it and drink it slowly while warm.

Tinctures. Ask your herbal shop to mix these in a bottle containing 50–100 ml (2–4 fl oz). Add seven to ten drops in a glass of cold or warm water, and drink slowly.

> ### CAUTION
> Herbal preparations should not be given to babies and children under three years old without expert supervision. For children between three and six years, add three drops; for seven-to-ten-year olds, add up to five drops.

Types of Touch

Massage is loving, caring, comforting, relaxing, soothing, invigorating, energizing and healing. To these ends, we use various techniques to massage in a variety of ways, depending on how we use our hands, the size of the area that is being massaged, and the depth of stroke. Some techniques encourage circulation and stretching, others pump toxins out of muscles, others relax the body. Following are the main types of touch used here.

EFFLEURAGE

Effleurage is derived from the French word *effleurer* which, broadly translated, means to 'touch lightly' or 'skim over'. It is a wide-area stroke performed with the palm of the hand and fingers; the aim is to massage in a rhythmic, smooth, flowing, gliding, stroking way. It is enhanced by the use of oil, and is an excellent way to begin and end a massage. Among its other benefits, effleurage creates an immediate sense of trust and relaxation between the person who is giving and the person who is receiving the massage.

Light effleurage promotes relaxation, alleviates pain and encourages sleep.

Deep effleurage improves circulation, stretches and relaxes tense muscles, helps lymphatic drainage and the elimination of waste products, and improves the elasticity of the skin.

Although effleurage is mainly performed with the flat palm of the hand in long regular strokes, it can also be practised with a cupped hand, by placing one hand on top of the other, and by using the tips of the fingers for 'feathering', a very calming and soothing technique.

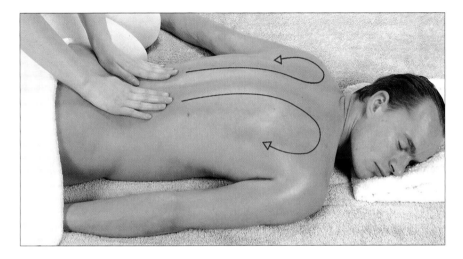

The flat-hand effleurage stroke is used on the arms, legs and the broad flat surface of the back. With the hands relaxed, always keep the momentum on the upward stroke, easing the pressure on the return movement. This relaxing, beneficial massage is superb for easing tensions and alleviating aches and pain.

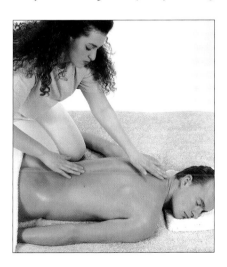

Feathering, achieved by finger-tip gliding over the surface of the skin, is a relaxing stroke that alleviates stress and tensions, and promotes calm. It is also used to finish a massage.

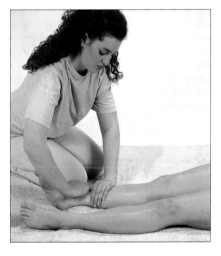

The cupped-hand effleurage massage is a light soothing stroke, useful for sensitive areas, such as calf muscles, and for improving circulation problems, such as fluid retention.

PETRISSAGE

The aim of petrissage is to stretch muscles in a deeper and more stimulating way than effleurage. It is a form of kneading, wringing and firm rubbing that can be practised with both hands together, with alternate hands, or with one hand on top of the other. The movements, used mainly on fleshy parts of the body, like the thighs, can be slow and deep or quick and energizing, gentle or firm. They relax tense muscles, releasing deep muscular contractions; revitalize tissues; improve circulation; and help to eliminate waste.

In kneading you use both hands alternately. The movements are a rhythmic squeezing which flow towards and away from each other. Wringing, most effective on the thighs and calves, adds a twist-action to the kneading. Keep the thumb close to the fingers. Push in opposite directions with each hand, squeezing the flesh between them. It is a flowing movement, but is deeper and more stimulating than kneading.

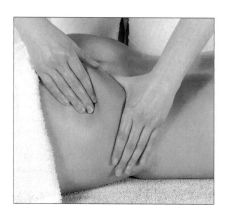

Kneading is a stimulating stroke used for releasing toxins, tightness and tensions from muscles and delivering a revitalizing supply of oxygenated blood to the areas being massaged. It is mainly used on the fleshy parts of the body, such as the thighs, legs and buttocks. Kneading is a variation of petrissage.

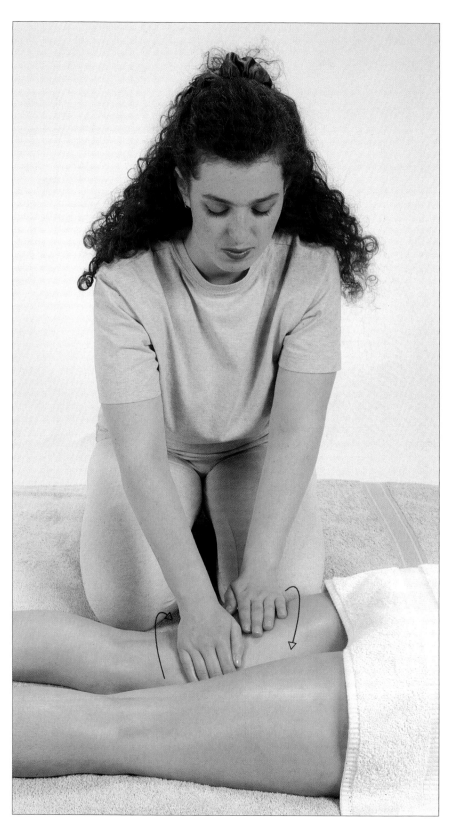

Wringing is a deeply stimulating massage movement, used on areas such as the thigh. It is achieved by positioning your thumb close to your fingers and using a gripping pull-and-release action on the muscles.

PERCUSSION

The three main forms of percussion are hacking, cupping and pummelling. The aim is to increase circulation, break down fatty deposits and revitalize tissues. The movements, which are mainly brisk and stimulating, but can be soothing if performed slowly, are most commonly used on fleshy muscular areas, such as the buttocks and top of thighs. They are never used on bony, injured or painful areas.

Keep your hands relaxed, maintaining a gentle flowing rhythm, using light springy movements. Watch for any discomfort in the person you are massaging. If a movement hurts, do not repeat it.

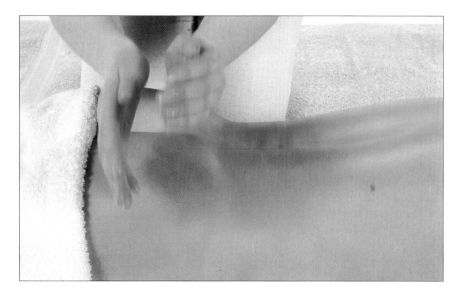

Hacking uses the sides of both hands alternately to deliver light, bouncy, chop-chop movements on areas such as the buttocks. It is essential to keep hands relaxed. This stroke stimulates the circulation and skin, and relaxes muscles.

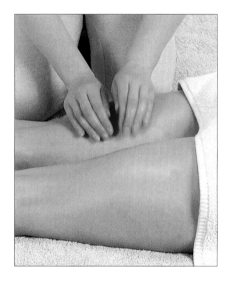

Cupping (see above) *is performed by arching the hands at the knuckles, keeping the fingers straight, and using the hollow part of the fists alternately in rapid up-and-down movements. It is excellent for treating the build-up of cellulite in the thighs.*

For pummelling, keep wrists relaxed, and make hands into loose hollow fists. Bounce the sides of the fists rapidly and lightly, alternately. It disperses tension and congestion, increases blood flow, and breaks up fatty deposits.

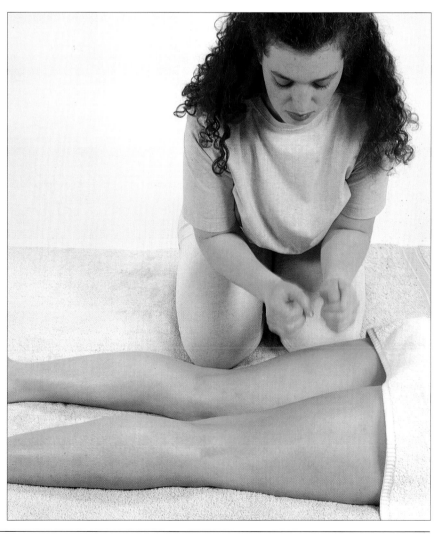

PRESSURE

These techniques are used for massaging smaller areas of the body, notably the muscles along the side of the spine and around the shoulder and buttocks area.

Thumb circling is achieved by tucking the fingers into the palm, or spreading the fingers for support, use the pads of the thumbs to press directly on the underlying muscles for a few seconds before releasing. To improve flow of energy and circulation, thumbs are used for applying a rolling circular pressure.

Pressure with the hands is used in the same way as pressure with thumbs, but here using the palm and heel of the hand.

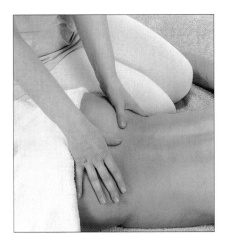

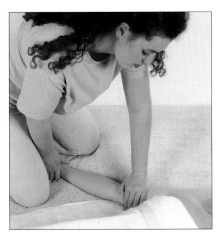

Thumb-circling pressure is used for massaging the back, tops of shoulders and calves. It is a deep, slow-rotation friction technique for toning up muscles and improving circulation.

Breathing in while leaning in on the palms of the hands to apply pressure, then breathing out as you release it, is a technique to stimulate and rebalance energy and alleviate pain.

ACUPRESSURE

Meridians and the acupressure points located on them are treated with thumb pressure. The pressure is applied using either a toning or sedating method depending on whether you wish to add to or disperse energy from a particular area.

To tonify (or tone) or increase energy, take a slow deep breath and as you breathe out press down with your thumbs for a few seconds. Keep the pressure firm and constant without hurting. Repeat three to five times.

To sedate or disperse energy, rotate your thumb in a clockwise direction (unless otherwise advised) in a gentle but constant manner for two or three minutes.

To treat mucus in the lungs, first use sedating pressure to disperse the phlegm and then tone to strengthen the lungs.

The bladder meridian runs down the back of body from the head, along the back of the thighs, to the little toes. Applying thumb pressure to this meridian on the leg area improves circulation and eases sciatica pain.

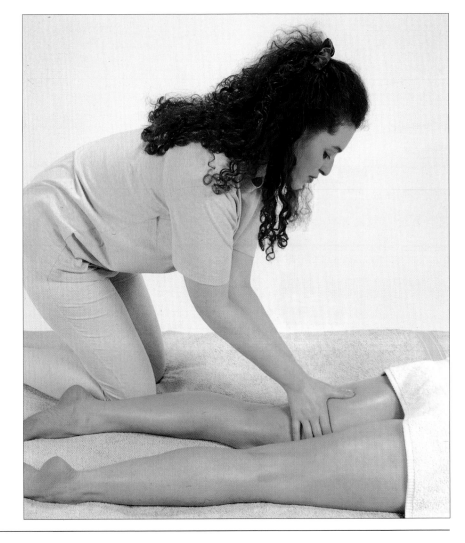

ARTICULATIONS

The aim of these techniques is to stretch and free any impeded joints and related structures, such as ligaments and adjacent muscles. By keeping the body supple, mobile, flexible and youthful, the onset of rigidity that is so common in ageing and all health problems related to the body's main structure of bones, joints, muscles and ligaments, is hopefully delayed or even avoided altogether. Oriental body therapy techniques and osteopathy make excellent use of articulations.

Supporting a limb, while applying pressure to stretch and articulate the part of the body that is being treated, forms the basis for many shiatsu techniques. This shiatsu stretch (see right) is used to free hip joints which are so prone to becoming inflexible as a result of arthritis, injury or ageing. The art is to stretch the joint gently as far as it will go comfortably without causing discomfort.

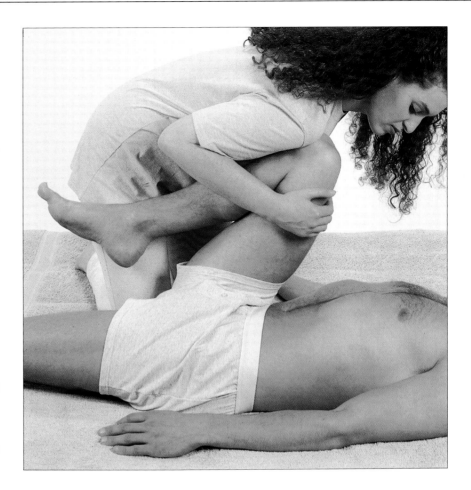

The Preparation

Creating the right state of mind, surroundings and atmosphere is as vital as the massage itself, so there are many important preparations to make before using therapeutic touch to soothe and heal.

The Room

Ensure this is clean and spacious, with a décor and ambience that calm the senses. Neutral colours, natural daylight or soft lighting are particularly conducive. Soothing, unobtrusive background music is often beneficial to both therapist and receiver.

The room should be warm but not stuffy. Remember that chilled muscles contract and tense up, so if the person who is receiving the massage feels cold, he or she will not be able to achieve the maximum benefit from the massage. It also helps to cover parts of the body that are not being massaged.

The massage surface needs to be firm, but not uncomfortably hard. A mattress or futon is fine, but you can, if you prefer, place a folded blanket, covered by a towel, on the floor. A purpose-built massage couch is, of course, a great asset.

The Massage Therapist

Giving and receiving a massage is an intimate activity, so sessions should be preceded by a bath or shower and tooth-cleaning. This applies to the person receiving a massage as well as the masseur. The therapist's nails should be short to avoid scratching or digging; hands well cared for; clothes loose-fitting; wrist watch and jewellery removed. The therapist certainly needs time and practice to build up stamina, and you should ensure that you do not bend or stoop in a way that creates aches and pains and back problems. Aim to keep your back fairly straight but not rigid, and turn from your waist rather than twisting your body in awkward positions. It is also very important to relax and to breathe deeply. This avoids your tiring and also enhances the effectiveness and sensitivity of your touch.

Keep conversation to a minimum – this is a time to relax. Talk before or after a massage.

During the massage, use your senses to monitor what the recipient is experiencing. Muscle contractions will alert you to any dis-

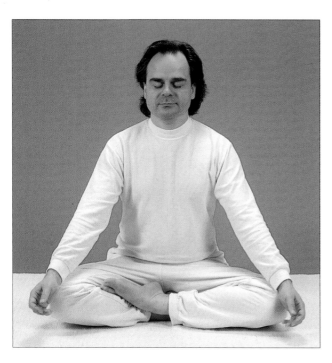

Meditation can be practised with your eyes closed in the position shown here, or by lying on your back with arms by your side, or when sitting upright in a chair with your hands resting on your knees.

It is practised to centre and free the mind by allowing thoughts, distractions and tensions to ebb and flow, without claiming the attention and disturbing the mind. To help, a mantra (sacred word) is often used. It is important to remember to breathe slowly and deeply.

Meditation is essentially for relaxing the mind and the body and freeing oneself from everyday worldly concerns and tensions.

comfort. Never repeat an action that hurts; always be guided by the recipient's expressions.

Creating the Right Frame of Body, Mind and Heart

Centre your mind on the person you are treating and the treatment that you are giving. Tense negative thoughts or a distracted frame of mind always have a direct influence on the quality of touch, which, as a result, becomes tense and unbeneficial.

A calm, centred frame of mind, heart and body ensures that both giver and receiver enjoy the maximum benefits from the session.

The following exercises will calm and recharge you with a positive peaceful energy that will put you in the right state before the session begins. This, in turn, will ensure that you give a truly healing and regenerating massage. The same exercises will recharge your 'batteries' after the session has ended.

Allow at least five to ten minutes for this relaxation exercise. Sit comfortably, or lie down on your back, and become aware of the muscles of your body. Are they tense or relaxed? To locate tensions, begin by concentrating your attention on your feet and gradually 'feel' your way up along calves, knees, thighs, pelvis, back, abdomen, chest, arms, hands, neck, skull, face to the top of your head. As you do this, note any tension and gently will the muscles to decontract and relax. If an area is particularly contracted, deliberately tense the muscles while, at the same time, taking a deep breath. Hold the breath for a few seconds and then exhale slowly, feeling the air leave you, and, at the same time, relaxing the deliberately tensed muscles. You can help this process by silently repeating words, such as 'Relax . . .', 'Let go . . .', 'Relax . . .', and so on. It will probably be necessary to repeat this procedure a few times.

We often do not realize, when concentrating, how very prone we are to holding our breath and making it shallow and irregular. This prevents essential oxygen re-energizing our bodies and plays a part in causing jerky irregular mas-

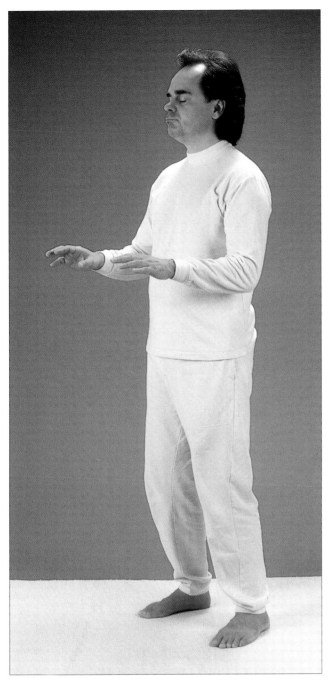

Stand with feet apart (see above) *parallel to the shoulders. Keeping your trunk straight and shoulders and arms relaxed, extend your forearms and hands to create a circle at the level of your navel. Relax your neck, tuck in your chin and flex your knees.*

Allow two minutes for each of the next three phases. Breathe from your abdomen and feel it becoming warm and vibrant with energy. Feel the energy rising and going to your arms and hands. Feel your hands becoming warm and vibrant.

Return to your normal posture, take a couple of deep breaths and allow your whole body to relax.

sage strokes. It comes about because we have been conditioned to believe, and subconsciously accept, that concentration is a form of effort that makes us tense up. A degree of tension is necessary for some daily functions, but is unnecessary for massage where the best results come from being attentive but essentially relaxed.

In the following breathing exercise visualize yourself lying in beautiful, harmonious surroundings – a sun-warmed beach, lapped by a calm blue sea and framed by a clear sky is an image that most people easily relate to. See and feel yourself lying on the sun-warmed sand, feel the warmth on your skin, and the presence of a light breeze. Give your attention to the harmonious sounds of the waves lapping in and out along the sand, and synchronize your breath with these. Breathe in and out slowly, deeply, and relax. This will release tensions and worries, and revitalize you physically, mentally and emotionally. Practise for ten minutes.

Life-giving Energy

Stand, sit or lie with your eyes closed or semi-closed, with both hands on your lap with palms facing each other about 25 cm (10 in) apart. Listen to your breath for a few moments until it becomes relaxed and harmonious. Then visualize a small dot of white-gold light emerging from your solar plexus (situated 8 cm/3 in from the end of your chest bone). Your regular and energizing breath, together with loving compassionate thoughts, will allow the white-gold dot to grow until it is a warm healing ball of light spreading through and encompassing a large area of your upper abdomen. Stay with this pleasurable sensation for a while and bask in its warmth and goodness.

Next, feel the light pervading your whole body, infusing it with warmth, well-being, health. Stay with this sensation for a while.

Then, feel its life-giving energy, as a ball of light, held in the palms of your hands. Feel its warmth and goodness. Relax, take a deep breath, slowly open your eyes.

You are now ready to begin the massage!

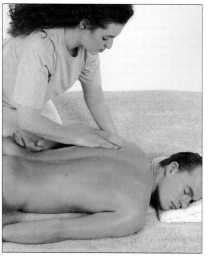

CHAPTER ONE: *A Healthy Back*

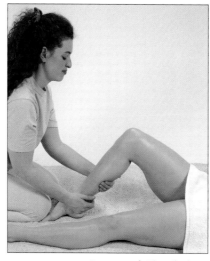

CHAPTER TWO: *Improved Circulation*

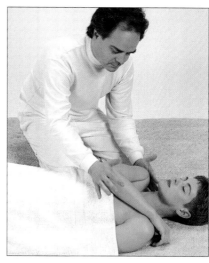

CHAPTER THREE: *Flexible Joints*

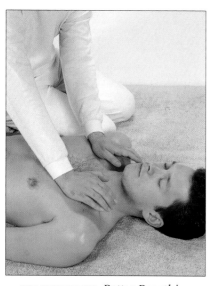

CHAPTER FOUR: *Better Breathing*

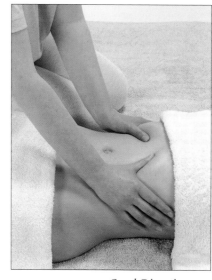

CHAPTER FIVE: *Good Digestion*

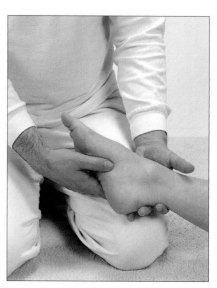

CHAPTER SIX: *Clean Water*

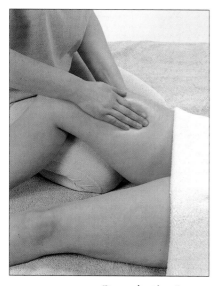

CHAPTER SEVEN: *Reproductive Issues*

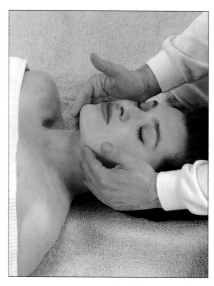

CHAPTER EIGHT: *A Clear Head*

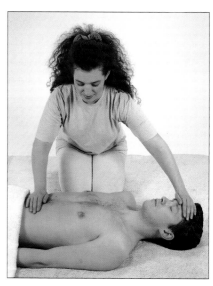

CHAPTER NINE: *Happy and Relaxed*

PART TWO
Caring for the Body

Part Two is presented chapter by chapter, so you can easily refer to the area of the body you wish to strengthen or where a complaint is to be eased. Caring for the body means our own bodies too and there is a valuable self-help section in each chapter. From Chapter One, A Healthy Back, possibly the most common area of discomfort, to the concluding Chapter Nine, Happy and Relaxed, each chapter is set out in an easy-to-follow pattern. There is an introduction to the body system, and a brief section on anatomy with a diagram, all valuable information for the therapist. Then common complaints, which can be eased through the use of massage and bodywork, are outlined and useful herbal teas, acupressure points and essential oils are given. Following are the top-to-toe techniques, the essence of the book and the most natural way to improve and maintain your well-being, always drawing together a range of massage techniques and natural treatments.

Put all the sequences together to form an all-over massage to promote general well-being and to keep the body in peak condition.

CHAPTER ONE

A Healthy Back

Massage and bodywork techniques relieve the symptoms of existing back pain, and help people who, so far, have a healthy back to keep it that way. Looking after the back and keeping it in good shape benefits the whole body and greatly enhances the quality of life.

Bad News

At least seventy per cent of people suffer from backache at some stage in their lives and, in about fifty per cent of these cases, the pain recurs within two years. Back pain is the most common cause of discomfort and disability in people under forty-five; and, with the exception of the common cold, is the main reason why people take time off work. Needless to say, this results in great financial losses both for the individuals concerned and for their employers. A stiff back hinders freedom of movement and the healthy functioning of nerves, and is a precursor to a surprisingly varied collection of problems, such as poor circulation, restricted breathing, premature ageing and arthritis.

Good News

The good news is that most backaches and pains can be prevented by keeping muscles and joints supple and mobile, and by learning how not to inflict unnecessary stresses and strains on the back and its component parts.

The aims of this chapter are to increase knowledge of how the back works, how to assist it with correct posture, and how to use the safest and most effective massage and self-help bodywork exercises to maintain it in tip-top condition. A combination of all of these will improve circulation and thus keep back

THE SPINAL STRUCTURE

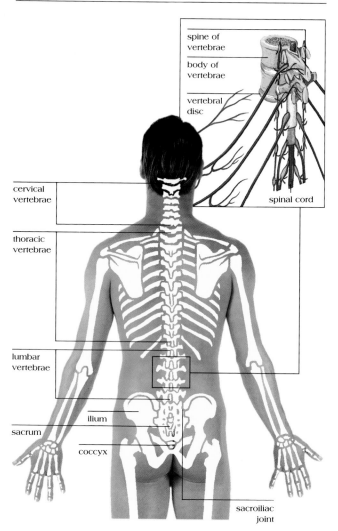

The spinal structure, commonly referred to as the spine (vertebral column), is the main support of the body, not only for the musculoskeletal system but also for the central nervous system which emanates from the spinal cord. Each pair of vertebrae is different from another, but each has extensions on both sides that arch protectively over the emerging nerves. Between each pair is a tough and resilient disc. Massage, exercise and correct posture all contribute to flexible healthy spinal joints.

muscles elastic, and the vertebral joints mobile and flexible and less prone to stress and injury.

Structure of the Spine

The spine (vertebral column) is composed of thirty-three vertebrae. There are seven bones in the neck, called the cervical vertebrae, which allow a great deal of movement, particularly rotation. Of these, the two uppermost, the atlas and the axis, make it possible for the head to move. Every time we look to one side, behind, or up or down, we are moving the neck.

There are twelve thoracic (dorsal) vertebrae in the middle of the back. In this area, however, because of the rib attachments, movement is more restricted.

In the lumbar (lower back) area there are five vertebrae, which are the largest and toughest. This is not surprising, since the lumbar area supports the rest of the trunk and has constant and considerable pressure applied to it.

Below the lower back is a single large bone called the sacrum which consists of five fused vertebrae. The sacrum supports the pelvis.

Finally there is the coccyx (tailbone) at the end of the sacrum, a rather small triangular structure consisting of four fused bones.

The spine has been called the spinal (vertebral) column, not only because of its shape, but also because of its functions. Firstly, it supports most body structures: the head is on top of it, the ribs and internal organs are suspended from it and the arms and legs, sometimes called the extremities, are attached to it. From the joints, formed by the vertebral bones of the spine, emerge nerves that regulate many bodily functions. As spinal problems commonly create pressure on a nerve, this, in turn, can affect other parts of the body. For instance, a lower back problem can cause numbness in the legs, and a similar condition in the middle spine can impair breathing or digestion.

The founder of osteopathy, Dr Andrew Still, fully appreciated the health implications that arise from this connection between the nerves of the spine and the rest of the body, and, at the turn of this century, many of his followers (osteopaths) believed that most illnesses could be treated by freeing the skeletal structure. That vision proved to be too optimistic, but some of the theories are, and always will be, valid. Certainly today's therapists can confirm this by treating the neck to improve headaches. By treating the lower back some conditions affecting the lower abdomen can be relieved.

In view of the spine's weight-bearing and supporting actions it is not surprising that it is prone to stress, strain and injury, and that backache and pain are such common conditions. Sadly, it is extremely rare for us to be taught how to look after our backs and, as a result, many unnecessary injuries are caused by thoughtless misuse and poor posture.

Ligament Problems

The bones of the spine are kept in line and bound to one another by ligaments – tough bands of fibrous tissue which can, through misuse, become weakened and overstretched. If a ligament is repeatedly injured, it is not easy to restore it to its original level of health; in some instances, it may remain weak, slack and vulnerable. For this reason, it is very important to treat any spinal misalignments, and to avoid abuses, misuses and postural errors – all factors that can over-stretch a ligament.

Disc Damage

Between each pair of vertebrae, with the exceptions of the sacrum and the coccyx (tailbone), there is a disc. This is a tough and resistant cushion that creates a space between the vertebrae, and acts as a shock absorber. Discs can thin with age, and can become inflamed or rupture with abuse. Incorrect posture, abrupt movements and damaged ligaments, as well as tense muscles and restricted joints, all put unnatural pressure on the disc.

When told they have they have a disc problem, the majority of people say they have 'put a disc out'. In reality, a disc does not come out

THE MUSCLES OF THE BACK

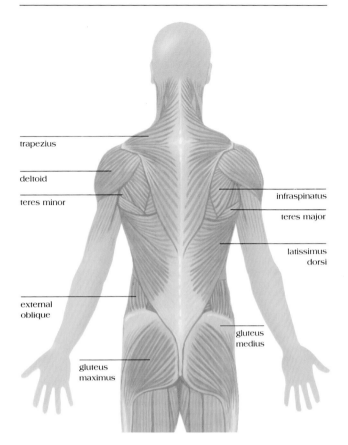

trapezius

deltoid

teres minor

infraspinatus

teres major

latissimus dorsi

external oblique

gluteus medius

gluteus maximus

Muscles of the back allow the movements of the spine and keep the posture upright. It is important to keep them supple and stretched.

of its place in the spine – it becomes herniated (swollen), presses on the surrounding structures such as nerves, or, in more severe cases, ruptures and spills fluid, severely affecting the surrounding nerves. For this reason, the nerves travelling from the spine to the feet, such as the sciatic nerve, can become inflamed and cause varying degrees of leg symptoms.

Rest, to avoid putting the disc under any further pressure, is essential for disc problems.

Muscle Strain

When stretched beyond their normal capacity, the muscles of the back can be strained and, when this happens, they protect themselves from further injury by going into a very painful contraction. The pain then increases when the person moves, especially if the offending movement is attempted again.

Massage, with its relaxing and stretching strokes, is very effective for treating muscle spasm, and for restoring the normal range of movements.

Cause and Effects

By now, you will appreciate that back pain has many possible causes and that the interrelated components can affect various structures. For instance, a muscular spasm can reduce mobility around a spinal joint which, in turn, creates pressure on a nerve, and so forth.

Essential Oils and Herbs

Back problems are usually accompanied by inflammation. This comes about when the body sends an extra supply of fluid and blood carrying antibodies and anti-inflammatory agents to counteract injuries, such as torn muscles or ligaments. All this defensive activity at the site of an injury can become a cause of discomfort itself and this, in turn, can create a sluggish circulation locally and excess fluid.

The signs of inflammation – the body's attempt to repair itself – are redness, swelling and heat; and the resulting pain can be quite unbearable.

MASSAGE CREAM

To 65 g (2½ oz) of aqueous cream, which can be purchased from your pharmacy, add 10 ml (2 teaspoons) of the following tinctures *(see page 18)*: marsh mallow root *(Althaea officinalis)*, chamomile *(Chamaemelum nobile* syn. *Anthemis nobile)*; 5 ml (1 teaspoon) of yarrow *(Achillea millefolium)*, and the following essential oils: 4 drops of lavender, 3 drops of chamomile, 2 drops of cypress and 2 drops of frankincense. Mix thoroughly and, during massage treatment, apply about 7 g (¼ oz) of the mixture to the affected area.

> ### MASSAGE OIL
>
> Use the following essential oils in the base oil. Mix 30 ml (2 tablespoons) of base oil with two drops of lavender, one of chamomile and one of geranium.
>
> During the acute stage of inflammation, if your therapist agrees, apply the oil daily and massage the back very lightly for a few minutes. When the condition improves, apply the oil on a once-weekly basis, using deeper massage strokes to hasten recovery and to prevent relapses.

Posture and Movement

People often claim that a bout of back pain started with a minor event such as a sneeze or a cough, or when bending down to pick up an object. It is quite true that, leaving aside degenerative and organic illnesses, the cause of sudden back pain often remains unknown.

Having said that, the following postural problems and case histories highlight some common causes of back troubles and pain.

Poor Posture

Many of us stand and sit in ways that are either too lax or too rigid, both of which can easily cause a range of back problems.

If you stand upright but relaxed against a wall you will feel that the vertebral column has natural curves. It caves in at the lumbar region (lower back) and comes out in the thoracic area (middle of the back). These natural curves should be constant in an upright straight back, but not exaggerated. Often, however, we slump our spine when standing and sitting, and hold our spine in a side-bend or slouched position, which in time creates a curvature of the spine. Such abnormalities can, of course, be congenital (present at birth), but too often they develop as a result of a too lax posture.

Other people are too rigid and, by holding themselves too tight, they reverse the natural curves of the spine and cause the lower back to stick out and the middle back to cave in. The classic example of this is the military posture.

Try to hold your spine as if you were standing against a wall, straight but relaxed. Be careful not to tense your shoulders, and maintain the natural curves in both the lower and middle back areas. Keep the weight distributed equally between the two legs and feet. This will give you an idea of how you should hold yourself most of the time.

Burst of Activity

An elderly person (but this could equally apply to a person of any age) has spent most of the winter relaxing in front of the fire, rarely taking any exercise or even stretching their back. By springtime, muscles are weak but tight, and joints are stiff and rigid. Come spring, there is a sudden burst of activity and a whole day is spent in the garden bending, stooping, twisting and turning to prepare the soil for new seeds. Suddenly, while bending down, the person experiences a painful spasm in the back and realizes that he cannot straighten up again, and eventually returns to the house doubled up in pain. The reason is simple: the sudden burst of activity has caused a muscle contraction or locked a joint in a very painful position.

Such an event could, of course, have been avoided by gradually preparing the body for renewed physical activity and then 'pacing' oneself by working for short periods that are slowly increased as the body becomes reaccustomed to the exercise. It is, in fact, a very good idea to precede activities such as gardening with a few minutes of stretching and bending exercises *(see pages 46–7)*. Also if backache, or more serious back problems, are to be avoided, all movements need to be performed with an awareness of the limitations that are imposed by age, infirmity or a sedentary lifestyle.

Choosing a Mattress

A couple save for some time to buy a luxurious bed and mattress. Having purchased it, they prepare themselves for blissful nights of sound sleep. This is not to be. Soon they both start complaining of back pain and restless nights. The new mattress is too soft, making them sink into a position that causes a curvature of their spines and places excessive stress on ligaments and joints.

The opposite can also be true. Some people think that, to keep their backs healthy, they need a very firm mattress, but the overnight change to a harder surface causes back pain.

A mattress should be fairly firm, but not so hard (or soft) that it causes discomfort.

Repetitive Stress Injury

People in occupations that involve constant repetition of one or a series of movements tend to injure their spinal joints. I often treat waiters, waitresses and dancers. Most right-handed waiters and waitresses carry their orders on the right hand, then twist from the right hip when serving. These repetitive movements often displace the right hip and lock the lumbar vertebrae.

Dancers engaged in modern ballet are a good source of income for osteopaths! Given that so many of their dance routines consist of sudden jerky movements and steps, this is not surprising, but many of the injuries could be avoided. The problem is that dancers often rehearse or perform without allowing sufficient time for warming-up exercises. If they did precede their dance routines in this way, they would be doing their musculoskeletal systems a great favour and would avoid – or at least reduce – many stress-and-strain injuries. All the self-help exercises can be used for warming up.

Domestic Causes

There are many other common causes of unnecessary back pain that could be avoided by remembering to take the following simple steps.

For example, when cleaning the bath, the all too common mistake of bending down and then twisting the back to reach the corners, frequently results in a lumbar joint locking and the lower back muscles going into spasm.

This is the spine saying: 'Don't do this to me'.

Likewise, the same common lock-and-spasm frequently occurs in the kitchen when we go up on tiptoes to reach something in an upper cupboard and twist while we are looking for it.

Indeed, twisted spinal movements, such as side-bending stretches in bath cleaning, are the surest and shortest route to back trouble.

Remember, if you need to reach something further away when bending, change your position so that twisting and turning the spine is unnecessary. If you need to pick up an object, do not bend from your waist with straight legs. Always bend gently from the knees, so that your legs, not your back, take the strain.

Acupressure Points

In Chinese medicine, the bladder meridian plays an important role, not just because of the organ it controls, but also because of its meridian (pathway). This meridian runs parallel on both sides of the spine all the way from the head down to the little toe. There are two portions of the bladder meridian running all the way down the back, but here I concentrate on the main part located two cuns (two finger widths) on each side of the spine.

Cuns. The width or length of various parts of the body are divided into measurements called cun(s). For example, there are twelve cuns between the elbow crease and the wrist, so the area is divided by twelve. An easy way to measure cuns: when the middle finger is bent, the distance between the first crease and the second is taken as a 'cun'. The breadth of the four fingers, close together at the level of the first joint from the knuckles, is three cuns.

A soothing massage along the bladder meridian of the back strengthens the spine and prevents spinal problems, and reinvigorates the organs. For example, massaging the bladder meridian in the upper back has a healing effect on the respiratory and circulatory systems; in the middle back it affects the liver and stomach; and in the lower back it benefits the intestines and the genito-urinary system.

BACK ACUPRESSURE POINTS

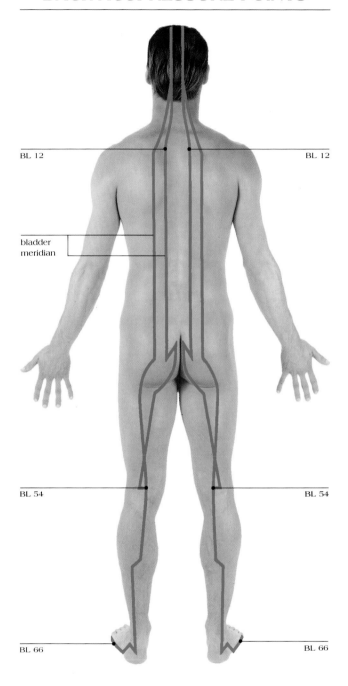

BL 12

bladder
meridian

BL 54

BL 66

The back and spine are central to the structure and functioning of the entire body, making the back acupressure points of great benefit. This is also the location of the bladder meridian which runs all the way down the back of the body either side of the spine from the head to the little toes. Massaging these points soothes and strengthens the spine and invigorates the other organs of the body. The specific back acupressure points are BL 12, BL 54 and BL 66 (see above).

This is consistent with Western understanding of how nervous reflexes work. For instance, early osteopaths based their approach on the fact that from each spinal joint nerves emerge which regulate many bodily functions.

Two cuns from each spinal joint along the bladder meridian, there is a point which acts on a specific organ. I describe only BL 12, BL 54 and BL 66 *(see below)*, because the other points require much more detailed knowledge which is beyond the scope of this book. Even so, if you press gently in succession from the top of the spine to the sacrum, you will find that this has a beneficial effect on all the organs.

You can also repeat the above sequence by pressing on both sides of each spinal joint for a few seconds. To recognize the spinal joints, feel along the spine with the tip of your index finger. You will easily feel the tips of the spine. In between each tip there is a lumbar joint (the space between two vertebrae), from where the spinal nerves emerge. The bladder meridian then continues all the way down to the foot along the middle of the back of the leg.

Bladder 12 (BL 12). This point lies on the bladder meridian two cuns away from the space between the second and third thoracic vertebrae. To find the first thoracic vertebra, ask the receiver to bend his or her neck and then rotate it to both sides. At the same time feel with your index finger the area where the neck joins the back. The last neck vertebra (cervical 7) moves with the rest of the neck, while the first thoracic remains still. BL 12 eases colds and fever.

Bladder 54 (BL 54). In the middle of the crease situated at the back of the knee there is a very important point called BL 54, which has two very beneficial effects. If, at every treatment, you massage this point on each knee for a couple of minutes it will help to resolve lower back pain, and will also cleanse and cool the blood, which is very beneficial for skin problems.

Bladder 66 (BL 66). This point lies at the junction of the little toe with the foot on the external or lateral side. Used for painful conditions of the bladder, such as cystitis. It can also soothe a sore and stiff neck.

Massage Sequence for the Back

There is nothing more delightful than a soothing relaxing back massage. In many ways the back is the best area to massage: it is a large, flat surface and is 'safe' to practise on because it is well protected by large muscles like the trapezius, which can be a site of tension. The back is a particularly good place to begin a full-body massage, but can also form an effective treatment in itself. Many of the back muscles help connect the torso to the limbs, so the benefits of this massage will be appreciated by the rest of the body as well. It is also the area of the body that people are least shy about having massaged, a good point for you to remember. The massage and bodywork techniques given here are a superb way to keep back muscles warm and elastic, to promote good circulation to the back, and to help to keep vertebral joints flexible, mobile and less prone to injury. A stiff back contributes to health problems such as arthritis, poor circulation, restricted breathing and premature ageing. What better reasons could there be to begin a massage right now!

1 *Effleurage is the favourite starting stroke for a massage session. Beginning with the back helps to relax the person being massaged and, at the same time, creates a feeling of trust and ease between the two people concerned.*

Ask your massage partner to lie face down with their arms at their sides, but slightly away from the body; then kneel alongside their hips so that you can reach from the base of the spine to the shoulders. Apply oil to the palms of your hands, rub it gently in, and position your hands at the sacral area (base of the spine). Breathe in and, while breathing out, glide your hands towards the shoulders always remembering to keep the spine positioned between both hands.

Having reached the shoulders, follow their contours with a gentle but even and firm pressure. Slightly relax the pressure and return towards the base of the spine, massaging the sides of the body. Keep your hands open, but in full contact with the body. It is important to perform effleurage with the whole hands not just with the fingers or palms. Return to the starting position at the base of the spine and repeat the sequence a few times. Reapply the oil when necessary.

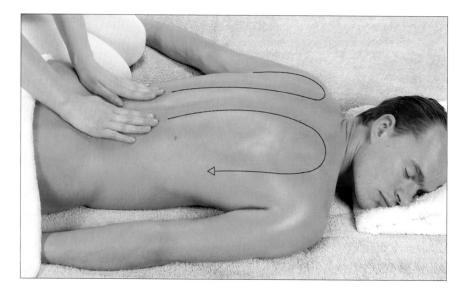

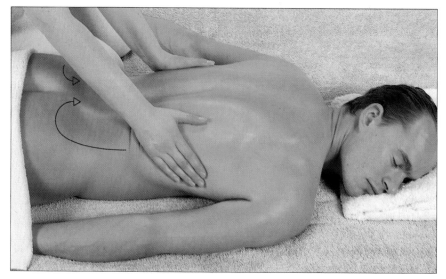

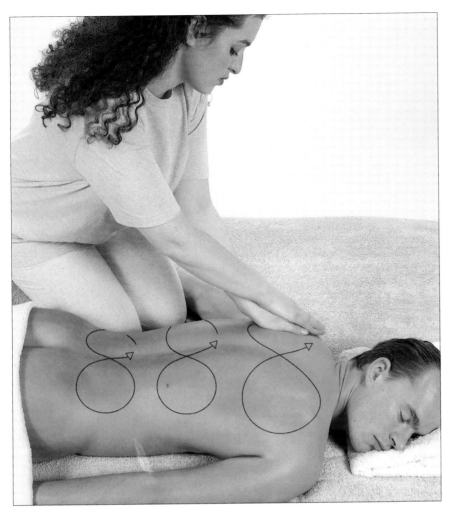

2 Position both your hands on top of each other on the shoulder closest to you. Draw a figure of eight from one shoulder to the next by drawing a zero (the first half of a figure of eight) on the area between the first shoulder and the spine; then draw the second half on the other side of the back. When crossing over the spine, soften the pressure. This whole movement should cover the upper third of the back. Repeat the same movement on the middle and lower back areas. Repeat, starting from the lower third of the back and return working up the back.

3 Place both your hands at the base of the spine and rub along the spine, using gentle pressure, towards the neck. Keeping your hands flat, use both hands alternately in a smooth rhythmic motion. As soon as one hand reaches the top of the spine, start at the base with the other. Repeat a few times.

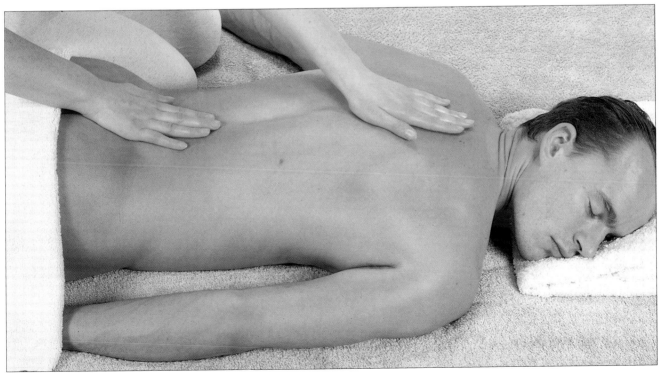

4 Locate the central gap between each vertebra and place one thumb on each side, 8 cm (3 in) away from it. As the person breathes out, press down gently but firmly with tips of thumbs, keeping thumbs straight. Release while he inhales and move to the next joint. Continue till the last lumbar (lower-back) vertebra. This revitalizes the spine, and the nerves emerging from it.

5 The small muscles immediately next to the spine easily become contracted and stiff limiting spinal movements and often leading to serious back problems. Place the heels of both your hands next to the spine and rub firmly, away from the spine, stretching the muscles. Repeat down both sides of the spine.

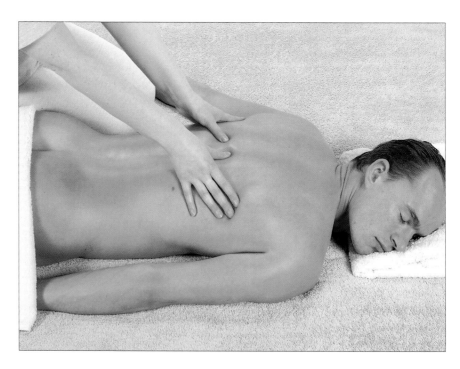

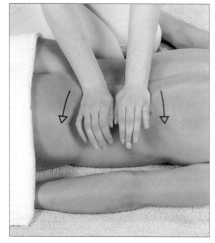

6 The following technique helps to free the thoracic (middle-back) area, and encourages better circulation to the chest improving the functions of all its organs.

Using your left hand, lift the left shoulder. This will widen the gap between the scapula (shoulder blade) and the middle-back area. Using the fingers of your right hand, massage the muscles around the shoulder blade towards the gap and gradually increase the gap still further. Tension and stiffness will slowly ease and 'give in' if this technique is used in a gradual, regular way. Repeat on the right shoulder.

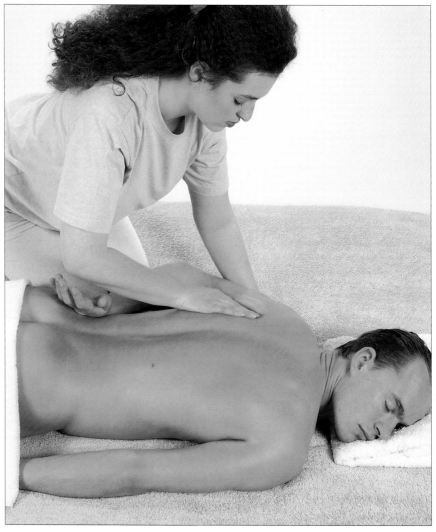

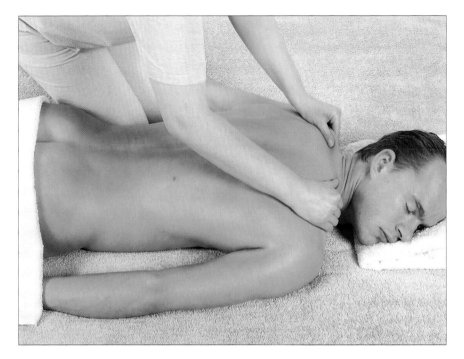

7 *Using both hands alternately and rhythmically, knead around the receiver's shoulders from the base of the neck to the acronium (bony tip where the shoulder ends and the arm begins).*

Massaging around the shoulder brings a great sense of relief as this area accumulates tensions and becomes stiff and sore. A large muscle, called the trapezius, covers the area ranging from the base of the skull across the width of the shoulders to the thoracic (middle-back) vertebrae. As a result, tension in the shoulders easily transmits itself to both the neck and the head causing symptoms such as headache, migraine and insomnia.

8 *Using your right hand for the right shoulder, and left hand for the left shoulder, press, applying a moderate pressure, at 2.5 cm (1 in) intervals, or a thumb's width, working inwards from the tip of the shoulders to the base of the neck. Always remember that the pressure should feel relatively pleasurable, and should certainly not hurt.*

The thumb's-width intervals that you should follow when applying the pressure from the bony tip of the shoulder to the base of the neck are shown below.

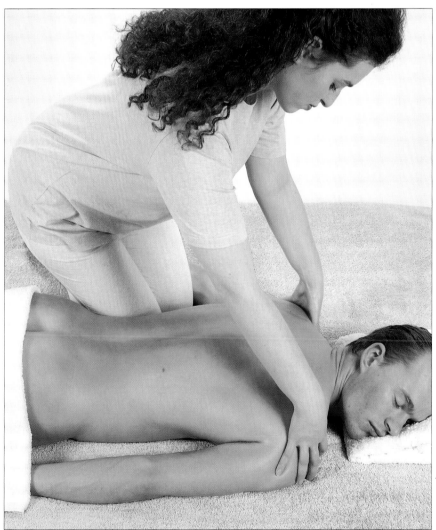

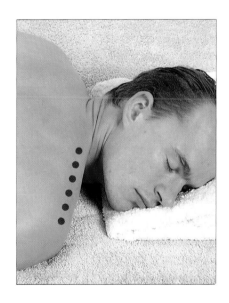

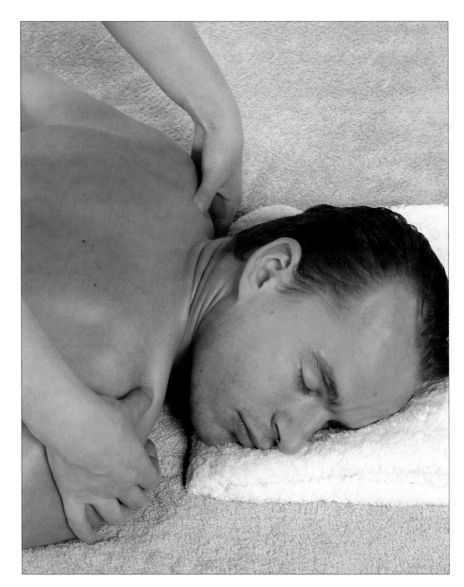

9 *This petrissage stroke is similar to step 7, but the motion is plucking the flesh rather than kneading and it is a deeper and more stimulating movement. Using both hands in an alternate, rhythmic, continuously flowing movement, just pluck and gently pull and stretch the flesh.*

10 *This technique follows the same pattern as the effleurage stroke used in step 1, but this time the massage is concentrated on the lower back area. Start the stroke with both hands together around the sacral area and upper buttock area. When you reach the waist area, follow the waist line, then, massaging with open hands, return along the back to the starting position of the upper buttock area. Repeat a few times.*

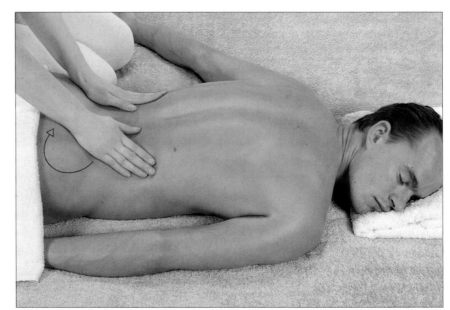

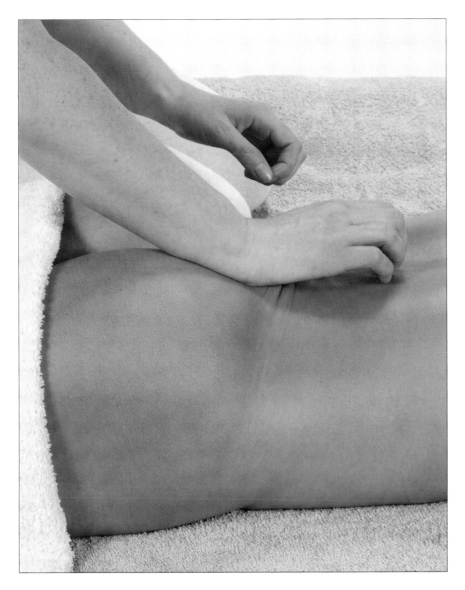

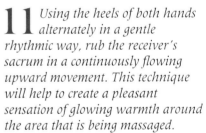**11** *Using the heels of both hands alternately in a gentle rhythmic way, rub the receiver's sacrum in a continuously flowing upward movement. This technique will help to create a pleasant sensation of glowing warmth around the area that is being massaged.*

12 *The sacroiliac joint is at the centre of many of our movements, such as bending, twisting and walking, and is prone to soreness and stiffness. The massage here consists of pressing with the thumbs and retaining the pressure on each spot for a few seconds. Working from the bottom part of the sacrum, massage your way around the pelvic bone all the way to the waist. Performing this technique once is generally sufficient.*

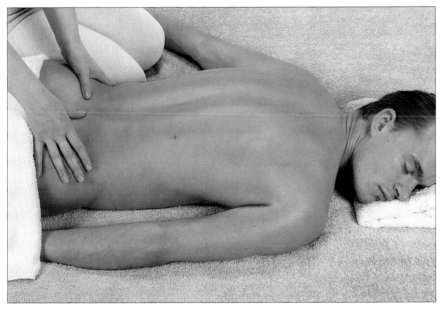

13 *Feel for the small dimples in the lower back on the sides of the sacral tip. This is where the sacrum and iliac (hip) bones meet. Starting from this area, which is called the sacro-iliac joint, use the heels of both hands to perform a petrissage stroke (see step 5) by rubbing away from the dimples and working your way to the bottom part of the sacrum.*

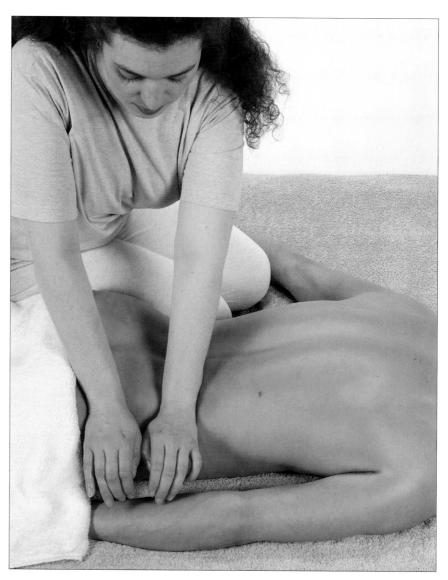

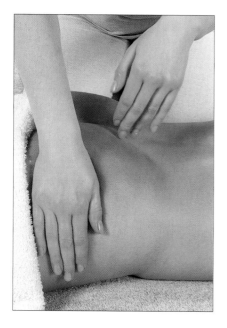

14 *Using both hands alternately and rhythmically, rub the buttocks in an upward motion (see above). This action will help to release the tension which so many people experience in this area.*

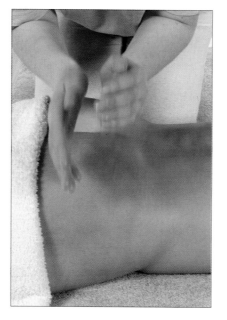

15 *Like all forms of percussion, this hacking movement should be gentle but firm and rhythmic. It is especially good for the buttock area and should be carried out over the entire area.*
  Keeping your hands loose and relaxed, hold them in a karate chop-chop position. Then, using the sides of both hands alternately, bounce on and off the skin of the buttocks with a hacking percussion movement.

16 *By now you will have noticed that some areas of the back accumulate more tension than others, and these areas feel particularly hard and stiff to the touch. With one hand on top of the other, use the heel of your lower hand to press and rub in an outward-going circle (see right) continue the massage until you feel the tension easing and subsiding.*

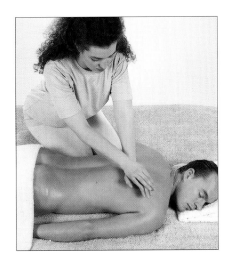

17 *Moving to a kneeling position above the head (see below), cup your hands (in a prayer position) and place over the spine. Breathe in and, as you breathe out, slide your hands down the spine to the lower back, then, opening your palms and keeping a firm contact with the flesh, return, massaging the sides of the body en route, to the starting position.*

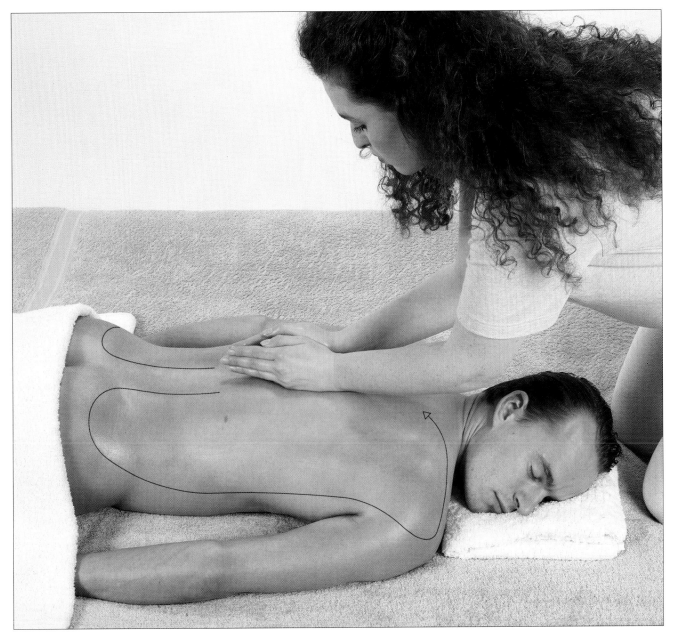

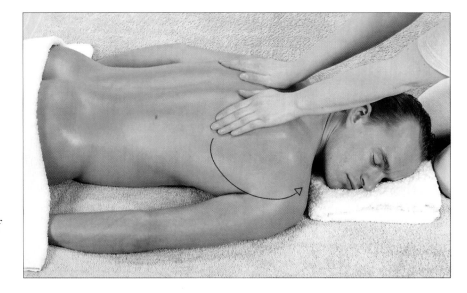

18 *Placing one hand each side of the receiver's spine, open the palms of your hands and, as directed in the previous stroke, retain a firm, unbroken contact with the flesh. Start the massage just below the base of the neck. Breathe in and, as you breathe out, massage down to the upper back* (see top right), *then return massaging the sides of the body. When you reach the shoulders, apply a firmer pressure and massage the shoulder blade muscles outwards towards the arms, almost, but not quite, tucking your hands under the recipient's shoulders* (see middle right). *Continue massaging with tonifying effleurage strokes to the base of the neck* (see below right).

Return to the original position below the base of the neck and start again. This time, as you breathe out, massage down to the middle back, completing the sequence as above.

Return to the original position and with soothing strokes massage down to the lower back, completing the sequence as above.

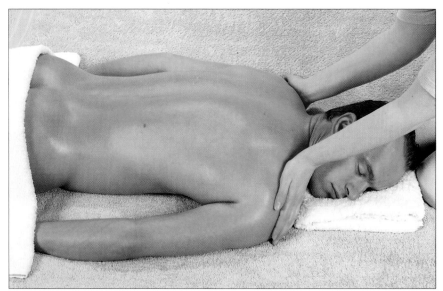

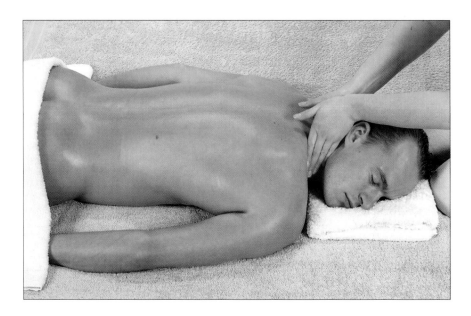

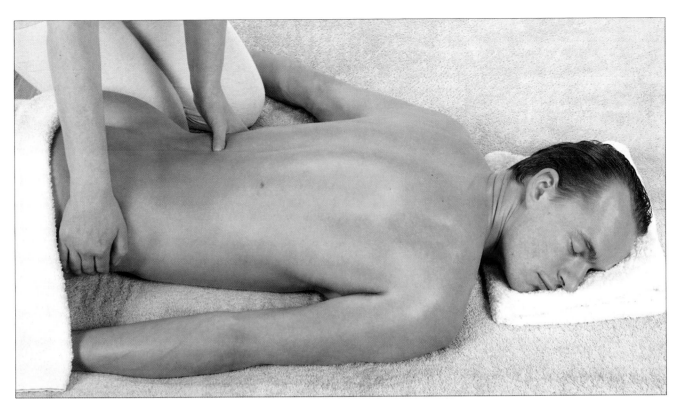

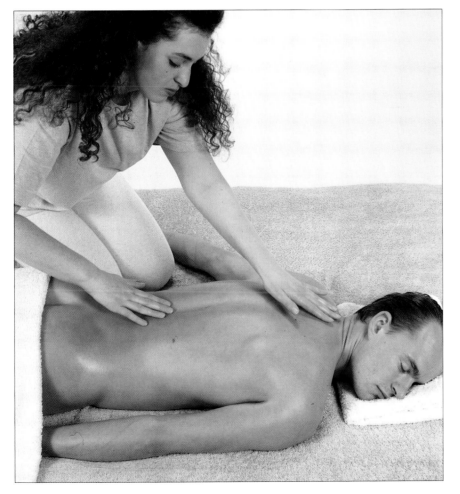

19 The following technique is very useful for freeing lumbar joints. Place your right hand beneath the ilium (hip bone) on the opposite side from where you are sitting. Place the thumb of your other hand between the first two lumbar (lower-back) vertebrae. Gradually lift the hip bone until you feel the lumbar joint move. Hold this position for a few seconds, then slowly release, and repeat the massage on the joints all the way down to the sacrum.

20 Most people find the following feathering technique very pleasurable and relaxing, but some find it ticklish. If this is the case, try a firmer, slower feathering movement, asking the person to breathe deeply in and out.

Feathering is an excellent way to end a back massage. Place the fingertips of one hand on the top of the back, just below the base of the neck, and, using feather-like touch strokes, travel rhythmically to the buttocks. On the return journey, use your other hand. Repeat.

Freeing Joints with Articulations

The following stretch-and-free techniques help to keep the body supple and flexible, increase the mobility of the entire spinal column, and are very useful for improving general posture, especially for people who are prone to round shoulders and a tendency to stoop.

Articulations should be performed very care-fully on children and older people and should not be attempted if there is acute pain. The therapist should perform articulations slowly and gently, always aware of the movement limitations of the recipient. The spine should never be forced beyond its reach. Encourage the recipient to say if there is any discomfort.

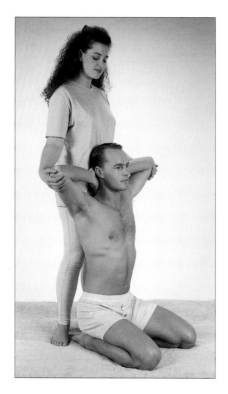

1 *The recipient can sit on his heels, or on the floor. Stand behind him, placing his hands behind his neck, elbows outstretched. Hold the elbows and place your knee behind his back. Ask him to breathe out and pull his arms further backwards while gently pushing your knee against his back to extend the spine. Repeat twice.*

2 *Same position, but no knee behind his back; as he breathes out, rotate his elbows and spine to one side. As he breathes in, return him to the starting position. When he breathes out, rotate him the opposite way. Repeat once.*

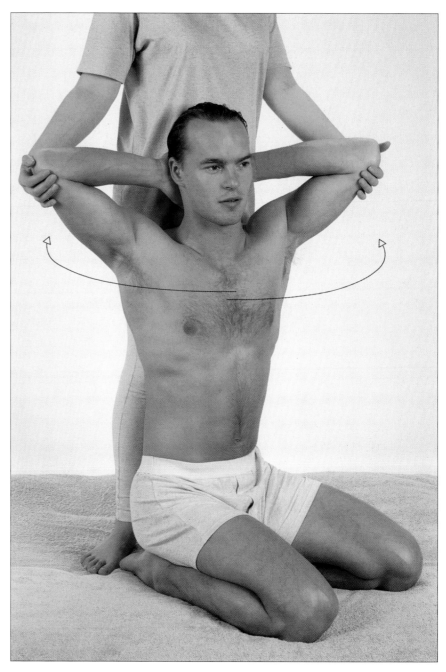

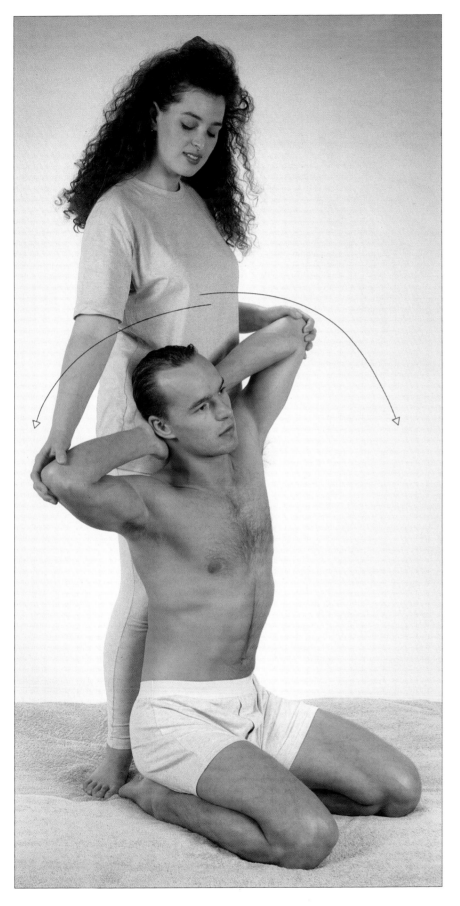

3 *Perform this technique while remaining in the same position, taking hold of his elbows and without placing your knee on the recipient's back. As he breathes out, bend his spine as far as it will comfortably go. Bend the opposite way. Repeat twice on each side.*

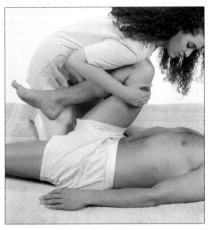

4 *Ask the person to lie on his back on the floor. Kneel alongside him, lift his leg, bend it from the knee and gently push it, as far as it will comfortably go, towards/against his abdomen. Hold the knee in this position for about ten to fifteen seconds encouraging the recipient to relax. Slowly bring it back to the floor. Repeat twice. Change sides and articulate the other leg.*

Self-help Exercises for the Back

A healthy spine is a very flexible structure. By various stretching, flexing, swivelling and rotating movements, it can extend and thus allow the whole trunk of the body to move freely upwards, downwards, backwards, forwards and sideways – to move, in other words, in whatever direction you wish.

Not surprisingly, considering how vital the spine is to freedom of movement, most forms of back therapy, through massage or exercise, aim to keep these movements unhindered and harmonious. Improvement to how the spine functions directly benefits the rest of the body.

The following self-help exercises ·are given with these thoughts in mind, and they will certainly help to keep your back flexible and healthy. They should be practised in a conscientious unhurried way, and the golden rule is never to force an action that is beyond your spine's natural range of movement. Any movement that feels comfortable and good is safe; any movement that is uncomfortable or painful should not be repeated. *(See also Self-help for Clean Water, page 103.)*

1 *Stand straight, arms hanging by your sides. Breathe in and, while breathing out, bend forward, arms reaching towards the floor. Remain for three to five seconds, breathing regularly, then return to the upright position. Repeat twice.*

2 *Place a hand on each side of your waist. Breathe in and, while breathing out, stretch from the waist backwards. Remain for three to five seconds. Return to the upright position. Repeat twice.*

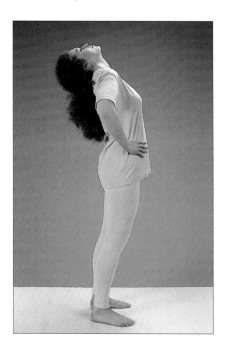

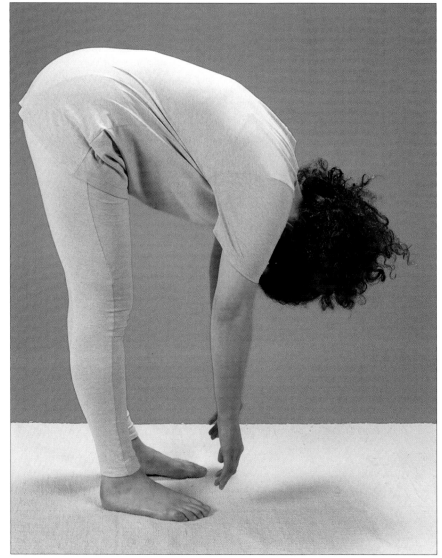

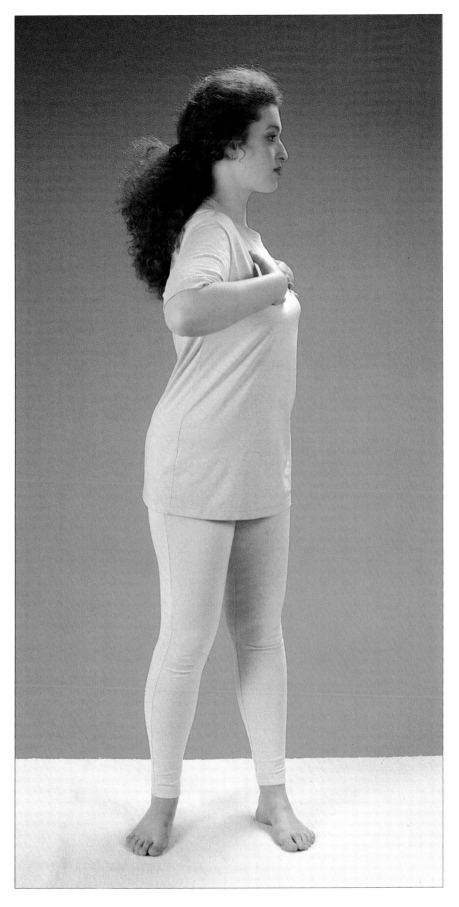

3 *Stand straight, legs slightly apart, and place one hand on each side of your chest. Breathe in and, while breathing out, rotate your trunk from the waist. Keep your head straight and look in the direction of the side to which you are rotating. Remain in this position for about three to five seconds always remembering to breathe regularly. Return to the centre and repeat this back exercise on the opposite side. Repeat the whole sequence two more times.*

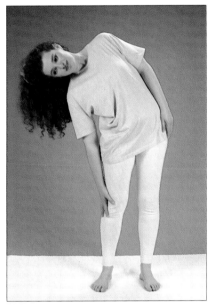

4 *Stand straight with your arms hanging by your sides. Breathe in and, while breathing out, bend to one side gliding your arm downwards towards your knee. Remain in this position for three to five seconds breathing regularly. Return to the straight position. Repeat on the opposite side. Repeat the sequence twice.*

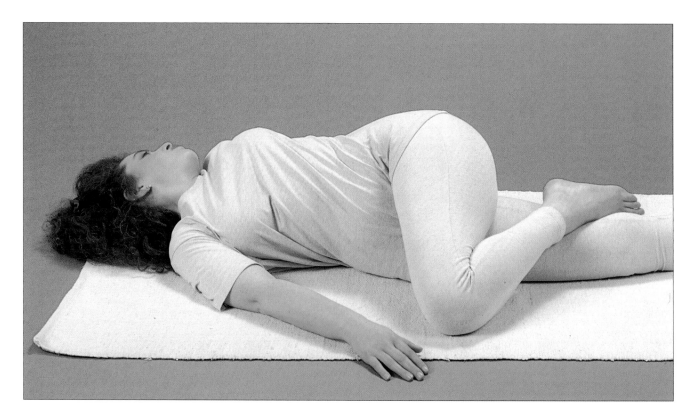

5 *Lie flat on your back, with your arms open at your sides in 'V'-like position. Place one foot on top of the opposite knee. Without raising your shoulders, begin to slowly twist your waist bringing your raised knee towards the floor. It is more important to keep the shoulders flat on the floor than to reach the floor with your knee. Reach as far as it feels comfortable. Remain in this position for a few seconds. Return to the resting position and repeat the movement on opposite side. Repeat once more on each side.*

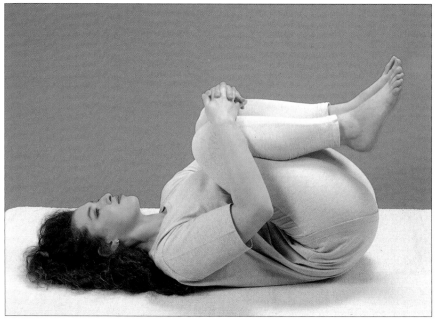

6 *Lie flat on the floor. Breathe in and, while breathing out, bring your knees towards your chest holding them with your hands. Remain in this position for a few seconds and then rock your body slowly back and forth for about one minute. Repeat this whole sequence once or twice.*

ALWAYS REMEMBER

● To breathe regularly.
● To perform slowly.
● Never to push the body beyond what is comfortable. The range of movement will increase with practice.

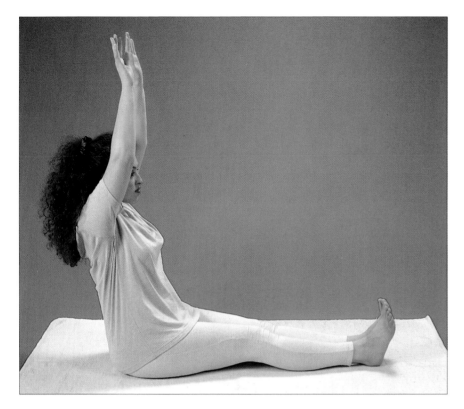

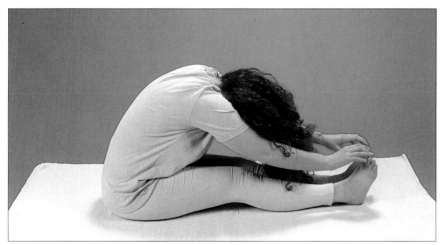

7 This exercise should be attempted in stages and never forced beyond what is comfortable. Sit on the floor with your back straight and your legs together. While breathing in, raise your arms above your head and, while breathing out, reach down and touch your toes, or ankles, or whatever part of your legs you can comfortably reach. Return slowly to the start position and try to touch your knees with your forehead. If this is difficult, bring your head and spine down as far as it is comfortably possible. Stay in this position for a few seconds breathing regularly. Return slowly to the start position and repeat once. You can gradually increase the time that you remain bent and the extent to which you can extend and stretch your spine, as your body slowly increases its range of comfortable movement.

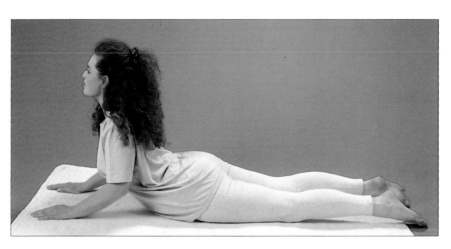

8 While performing this press-up exercise, visualize a cobra effortlessly raising its body from the ground. Lie on your stomach with both your hands level to your shoulders and your elbows bent. Breathe in and, while breathing out, use your hands to slowly but steadily raise the top half of your body, arch your back, look up and, when comfortable and without straining, remain in this position for a few seconds. Repeat this sequence one more time.

Reflexology

The therapy, known as reflexology, uses thumb pressures all over the foot to treat tensions and common ailments in other parts of the body. This is possible because the sole of the foot contains thousands of nerve endings (reflex points) that have their opposite ends sited all over the rest of the body. Massaging the foot in either a soothing and relaxing or stimulating way, according to need, can have an overall physical and mental balancing effect.

Because the foot is believed to be a map of the whole body, reflexology is also used for diagnosing weaknesses and health-related problems in any bodily system or organ. This is achieved by the reflexologist detecting crystalline deposits under the skin at the many reflex points of the foot. The aim, then, is to use massage to disperse the deposits and thus encourage the body's self-healing processes. Neck tensions, for example, are treated by using the thumb to massage in a circular way around the 'waist' reflex point of the big toe.

Reflexology is certainly delightfully relaxing, and thousands of people have confirmed that it has had an amazingly beneficial effect on their general health and well-being.

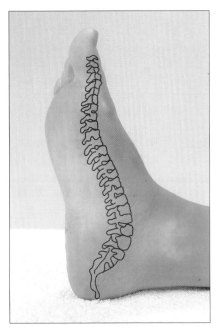

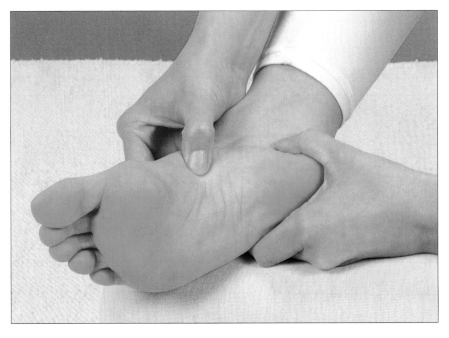

This is a simple introductory, and very effective, reflexology exercise. Unless the skin of the feet is exceptionally dry, oil is not usually used for foot massage. When it is, a tiny amount is sufficient. First, hold your foot and study the 'line' that runs along the big-toe side of your foot all the way to the turn of the heel. The 'line' is positioned in the part of the flesh where there is a skin change between the upper foot and the sole. Visualize a 'neck' around the big-toe area, and a 'hip' and 'sacral' area at the heel. The end of the lumbar area is where the heel starts. Having done this, you are now in a position to divide and locate the various areas of your foot that correspond with the various areas of your spine and hip (see above left). Using your thumb to rub firmly in a circular way, work down the line of your foot concentrating on any part that corresponds with any particular problem area of your spine (see above). (See also The Spinal Structure diagram on page 28.) Over a period of time, this thumb massage will gradually help break down crystalline deposits at the relevant reflex points on the sole of the foot. As your self-help reflexology slowly breaks down and disperses these deposits your body's self-healing processes will be promoted.

CHAPTER TWO

Improved Circulation

The circulatory system consists of the heart, the blood vessels, the blood itself and, to a certain extent, the lymphatic system. It is vital to the health and survival of every single part and cell of the body, and the elimination of waste. Poor circulation can starve certain regions of the body of vital nutrients, giving rise to health problems. Massage, using life-enhancing essential oils, and self-help exercises are both superb ways to maintain good health and improve poor circulation.

The Circulatory System

The heart, which performs the dual functions of sending out life-preserving oxygen-rich blood and receiving back blood laden with impurities, is best described as two simple muscular pumps that beat as one, continuously and rhythmically contracting and expanding in order to send blood to and from the lungs to the furthest parts of the body.

The function of the first and strongest pump (left side of the heart) is to receive the oxygen-rich blood from the lungs, and then pump it out, with a strong enough push, to carry it to every part of the body.

The blood, having been circulated to deliver most of its oxygen, is then returned to the right-hand side pump, which then pushes it through to the lungs to dispose of carbon dioxide and pick up more oxygen.

Once the blood is in the lungs, the waste and the waste gases are eliminated by breathing out, and exchanged for more oxygen by breathing in. The oxygen-rich blood then continues to the stronger left-side pump to start the circulatory journey all over again.

These complex activities happen almost simultaneously: as the left side of the heart contracts to pump blood to all the tissues throughout the body, the right side contracts to pump blood to the lungs.

The actual job of propelling blood through both sides of the heart is carried out by the solid muscle of the heart walls, the valves which continuously open and shut, and millions of individual muscle cells.

The whole cycle for the total volume of blood to circulate can take, while at rest, approximately one minute; during activity and strenuous exercise, it increases to between two and six times a minute.

Arteries, Veins and Capillaries

The dual-function heart pump, which begins and ends each distributing cycle of the blood, is backed up by arteries and veins. The arteries are red thick-walled muscular tubes which carry the oxygen-rich blood away from the heart, passing it on, through blood vessels, to the head and all the way down to the toes. The thin blue vessels, called veins *(see diagram page 52)*, transport the deoxygenated blood with the waste gases from the cells back to the right side of the heart in an upward movement.

Because both the arteries and veins are too large to carry the blood directly to and from the cells, there are also microscopically thin extensions called capillaries, and every part of the body has its own capillary system. The arteries and veins transport; the capillaries carry on the circulation passing oxygen and nourishment to every cell in the body, and taking waste gases from the cells back into the blood. The term 'broken capillaries' refers to the tiny red threads most commonly seen on the face and legs.

51

CIRCULATION OF BLOOD

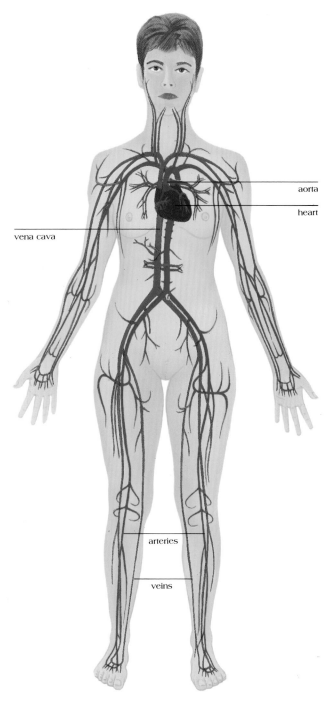

The heart pumps out – circulates – blood through arteries (shown red) into ever decreasing blood vessels until it reaches small capillaries that pass oxygen and nutrients to the cells, and wastes and carbon dioxide back into the blood. The blood returns to the heart along blood vessels, known as veins (shown blue) and then on to the lungs for disposal of waste gases.

Broken capillaries can be caused, for example, by corticosteroid drugs, a physical blow, and vitamin C deficiency.

Blood

Every part of the body depends on a continuous flow of blood. The vital body fluid has several essential functions.

Firstly, blood is a transport system picking up oxygen from the lungs and delivering it to the tissues by means of red cells. Most activities that take place inside the cells are totally dependent upon oxygen, which ensures their survival and continual regeneration.

Secondly, blood transports and delivers the white blood cells, which are the vital components of our immune system. This system defends us against invasion by bacteria, parasites and other harmful substances. The blood is also constituted so as to prevent uncontrolled haemorrhage when an injury occurs.

Thirdly, blood picks up from our digestive system the nutrients which are produced by the food we eat, and carries off waste products to the kidneys and liver for removal and neutralizing. It does the same with certain hormones, which exert control over many of the body's physical and chemical activities. The blood

---

BLOOD PRESSURE

This refers to the pressure exerted by the blood as it flows through the main arteries.

In the normal course of events, blood pressure rises and falls according to the demands being made by the body when it is active or inactive.

If, as a result of ageing, poor diet, or nervous and emotional tension and stress, the arteries are constricted in any way, the blood has to increase the pressure it exerts in order to circulate. This condition is described as high blood pressure.

A drop in blood pressure, which can make us giddy when standing up too quickly, is described as low blood pressure.

With each heartbeat, the blood pressure wave is transmitted along the arteries, and this is described as the pulse.

THE LYMPHATIC SYSTEM

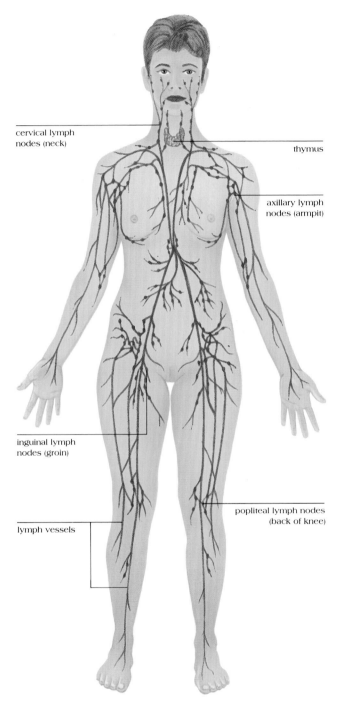

cervical lymph
nodes (neck)

thymus

axillary lymph
nodes (armpit)

inguinal lymph
nodes (groin)

popliteal lymph nodes
(back of knee)

lymph vessels

The lymphatic system, which is dependent on muscular contraction, works through valves and lymph vessels. The lymph (extracelluar fluid) which accumulates and filters nutrients and waste products, circulates through lymph nodes (glands). These nodes, aided by lymphatic organs, manufacture white blood cells. This system is vital to immunity against disease and repelling infections.

collects the hormones from glands and delivers them to the cells.

Fourthly, blood distributes heat from the centre to the periphery of the body. This is essential in order to maintain body temperature and a stable internal environment, in which the tissues of the body can function efficiently.

The Lymphatic System

This is best considered as a subsidiary of the circulatory system because, although it has its separate channels, the lymphatic system, which carries a fluid containing nutrients, oxygen and white blood cells to body tissues and waste matter away, closely follows the same pathways as the circulatory system.

The lymphatic system is widely distributed within the body in numerous lymph nodes, commonly referred to as lymph glands. The tiny transparent lymph vessels, which carry the lymph, resemble veins. They also help to manufacture and store antibodies that are so vital for neutralizing or destroying harmful micro-organisms.

By conveying lymph around the body, the lymphatic system plays a vital part in the maintenance of the immune system, helping to prevent and fight infection.

We usually become aware of the lymphatic system when lymph nodes (glands) become swollen – particularly in the neck, armpits, groin and behind the knees – due to over-activity or infection.

Because the lymph fluid is not circulated through the action of the heart, exercise and massage are very useful ways to maintain a healthy flow and enhance well-being.

Common Complaints

Complaints of the circulatory system can range from the uncomfortable, such as chilblains and cramp, to the more serious, such as high blood pressure. Massage is valuable in helping to ease some of the following complaints.

Chilblains

This poor circulation problem is always at its most distressing following exposure to winter cold spells. It is characterized by localized swelling and inflammation of the hands, fingers, feet and toes, accompanied by intense itching and burning sensations.

All circulation-improving massages help to avoid or treat chilblains, but the feet and hand massages are particularly helpful. The essential oils of marjoram or rosemary stimulate the circulation; and chamomile and lavender help to ease the inflammation.

Cramp

This painful muscular spasm can occur during or after exercise; or following repetitive movements; or even during the night. It is caused by a build-up of lactic acids and other chemicals in the muscles or the loss of sodium salts through sweating or feverish infections.

Cramp is relieved by massage, using gliding and deep kneading strokes, and self-help stretching exercises, which increase circulation to the painful part, often experienced in the calf muscles. Use the essential oil of lavender.

High blood pressure

When blood reaches the parts of the body that need it, it has to be at the right pressure. Too much pressure (high blood pressure) can have an adverse effect on a variety of different organs and functions of the body. If this condition is caused mainly by stress and tension, massage certainly helps by relaxing the muscles and allowing the blood to flow more freely.

The main aim when treating high blood pressure is relaxation. Massage, using gentle, rhythmic strokes, concentrates on the hands *(see page 63)* and feet *(see page 58)*, and the neck, head and face *(see page 117)*. Use essential oils, such as lavender, neroli, chamomile or orange peel.

Oedema

This problem, more commonly referred to as fluid retention, is often created by poor lymph drainage, and is frequently accompanied by

---

> ### HERBAL TEAS TO IMPROVE CIRCULATION
>
> Relaxation and breathing exercises help to improve circulation, as do the following herbal teas: ginger root *(Zingiber officinale)*, hawthorn flowers *(Crataegus oxyacanthoides)*, lime flowers *(Tilia europaea)*, rosehips *(Rosa canina)*, and rosemary *(Rosmarinus officinalis)*. Infuse 5 mg (1 teaspoon) of your chosen herbs in a cup of hot water for five minutes and drink while warm. WARNING. Avoid rosemary if you have high blood pressure.

inflammation and swelling. It can also be caused by rheumatic and arthritic conditions; ageing; and injury. Both 'water on the knee', or swollen ankles, for example, are really oedema.

Massage with the diuretic essential oils of lavender, fennel or juniper.

Poor circulation

When this is characterized by excessively hot and red extremities (hands and feet), treat with the massages given in this section, using 30 ml (2 tablespoons) of base oil to which you add one drop each of cooling essential oils, such as lavender, vetiver and cypress.

When characterized by cold and pale extremities, particularly common during winter months, treat with the massages given in this section, adding one drop each of rosemary, ginger and cypress to 30 ml (2 tablespoons) of base oil. If you also suffer from high blood pressure, avoid rosemary.

Vitamin supplements, such as vitamin C, vitamin E, bioflavonoid (vitamin P), and rutin (a glycoside obtained from buck-wheat), help to improve poor circulation. Ask your doctor or health shop to advise you on the correct dosages for your condition.

Swollen ankles

This fluid-retention problem is exacerbated by a sedentary lifestyle; travelling, especially when legs are confined; premenstrual tension; pregnancy; ageing, particularly among the inactive; or injury, such as insect bites and sprains.

ACUPRESSURE POINTS

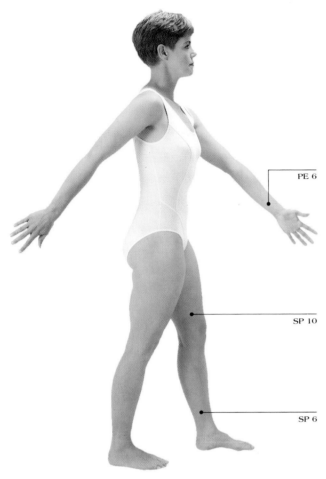

These acupressure points are used to promote better circulation by increasing the blood flow. They also help to strengthen the circulatory vessels, that is the veins and arteries. The points can also help to strengthen the quality of the blood itself by increasing the oxygen supply and assisting in the removal of toxins. Some are very specific in their benefits, for example easing cramps.

Massage can help by encouraging the flow of lymph which aids the drainage of fluid at extremities of the body. When massaging, use light effleurage (stroking) on the area from the foot to the knee; this is a perfect treatment for helping the circulation to flow back up the legs to the heart. Continue the massage for a minimum of thirty strokes, also including if possible the front-of-legs' massage sequence shown on pages 60 and 61. Choose from diuretic essential oils, such as juniper and fennel, and circulatory ones like cypress or lavender. Avoid the use of juniper if you are pregnant.

Varicose veins

These enlarged, blue, twisted veins are most commonly seen on the backs of the calves and the insides of the leg. They are made worse by poor circulation and prolonged standing. Aching, swelling of the feet and itchy skin results.

Massage helps to prevent varicose veins by stimulating and encouraging good circulation. If they already exist, do not massage directly over the top of the varicose vein area. Instead, massage the feet and legs using light effleurage (stroking), and avoiding petrissage (squeezing, kneading, wringing and pummelling) strokes. Lavender, vetiver and cypress are perfect oils for this massage.

Acupressure Points

Those that improve circulation are Spleen 6 (SP 6), Spleen 10 (SP 10), and Pericardium 6 (PE 6), all described here.

Spleen 6 (SP 6). From the tip of the inner ankle bone (malleolus), it is located three cuns up next to the shin bone (tibia). It is a point with varied applications, but should be used carefully on women who suffer from excessive menstrual flow. It should not be used on pregnant women. This point promotes circulation.

Spleen 10 (SP 10). Find the superior (top) ridge of the knee, and then move to the side of the ridge on the inner leg. The point is two cuns (finger widths) above this. SP 10 increases and promotes good circulation, cools and cleanses blood, and is helpful for treating skin diseases.

Pericardium 6 (PE 6). Find the middle of the wrist crease; this point is two cuns above it. When you flex and tighten the forearm, you will see two tendons running in the middle part of the inner arm. PE 6 is in the middle of those two tendons. This point is very good to release anxiety, particularly when accompanied by a sense of tightness in the solar plexus, commonly called 'butterflies'. Good to soothe pain, cramps and general tension.

Massage for Improving Circulation

Massage is a wonderful way to maintain and improve the circulatory system. It increases the supply of oxygen and nutrients, which, in their turn, circulate to strengthen and regenerate the whole body.

The alternation between pressure (squeezing) and relaxation (releasing) that massage exerts on muscles, creates a pumping effect that encourages lymph drainage and the elimination of toxins, and strengthens the heart for maintaining good circulation.

Without a doubt, tense muscles and nerves, congested organs, and restricted joints all add up to poor circulation. The following massages concentrate on the legs and arms, places where circulation can easily slow down.

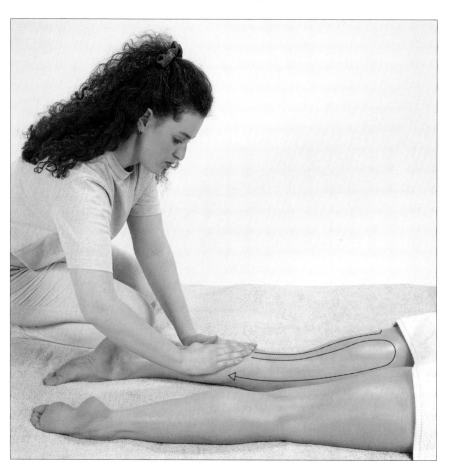

1 *Kneel alongside the feet of the person you are massaging and place both your hands flat on the lower leg (see right). Breathe in and, while breathing out, perform an upwards effleurage stroking up the centre of the entire leg. When you reach the top of the thigh, return to the starting position by massaging the outside of the leg, using your palms and fingers. Repeat twice. Make sure that you move your whole body as your hands travel up the legs, so that you can easily reach the upper thigh.*

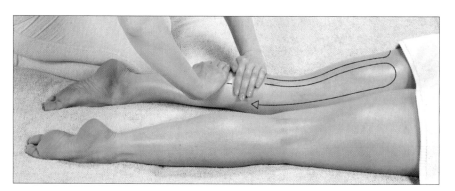

2 *Cup your hands around the lower leg, fingers pointing in opposite directions. Create a slight pressure by leaning in from your shoulders and use a gliding stroke up the leg, avoiding pressure on the back of the knee. At the top of the leg, open your palms, and kneel up, leaning into the thigh. Curving your hands around the thigh, draw them down the outer leg. Repeat twice.*

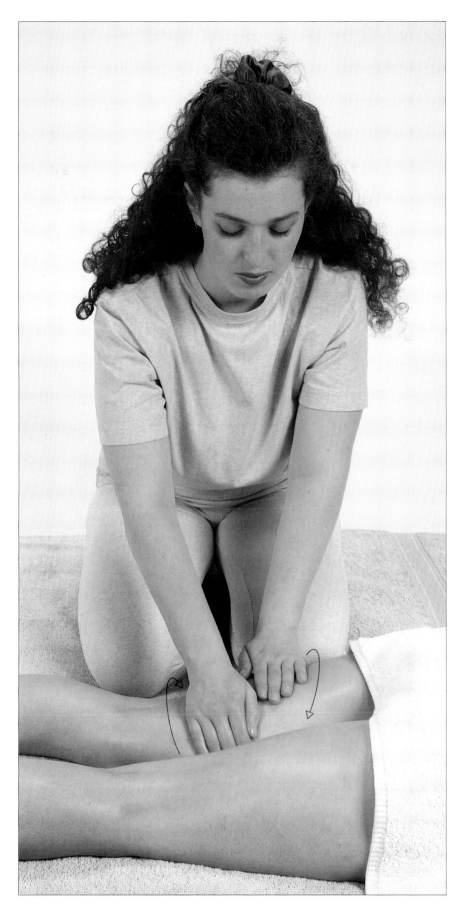

3 *Position yourself at right angles to your massage partner* (see left) *facing the backs of the knees and the upper thighs. Place your hands side by side over the nearest thigh and, leaning into one hand, perform a petrissage wringing movement squeezing the flesh between your hands as they pass each other. Work rhythmically over the whole thigh massaging all the way down to just above the knee line, then moving back to the top of the thigh. Use firm pressure but be careful not to pinch too hard, causing unnecessary pain.*

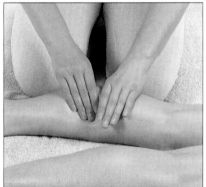

4 *From the same position, kneeling at right angles to the recipient, lean in from your shoulders to create a slight pressure and, using both hands alternately, knead the calf area by picking up and pulling the flesh and muscles between finger and thumb. Do not perform this stroke if there are broken capillaries (blood vessels) or varicose veins on the leg area.*

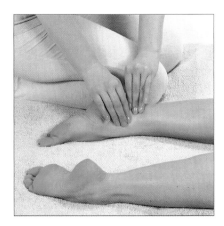

5 *Position yourself alongside your partner's feet* (see above), *and use the fingers of both hands to gently pinch and pull the flesh surrounding the ankle area.*

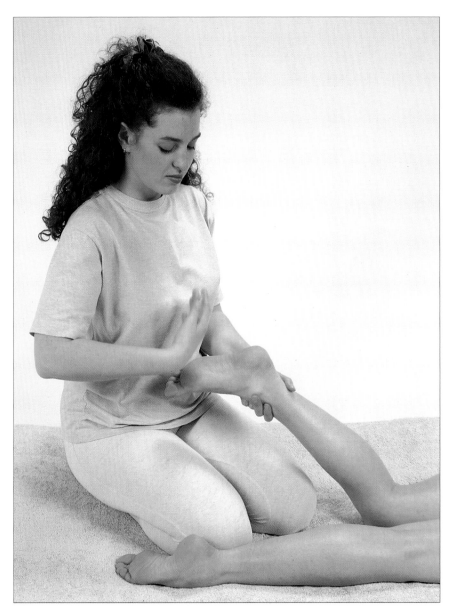

6 *Firmly supporting the foot* (see right), *use the back of your hand to make a quick, light, hacking movement on the sole. This invigorating technique stimulates the entire circulatory system, makes a person more alert, and also increases their vitality.*

7 *Holding the recipient's foot steady at the ankle* (see right) *use the palm of the hand to make rapid, invigorating rubbing movements on the sole of the foot. This technique takes both practice and sensitivity to apply just the right amount of pressure and speed to stimulate the circulatory system while avoiding tickling.*

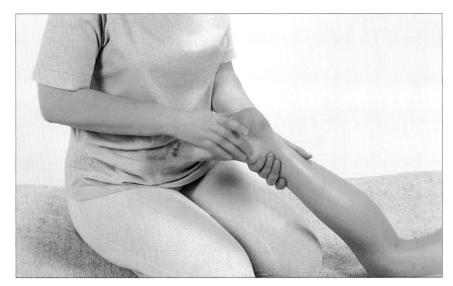

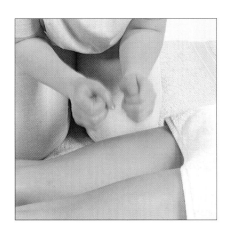

8 *Keeping your wrists flexible, and using both your hands as loose relaxed fists (see right), pummel the back of the thigh with light, bouncy, stimulating movements. Do not perform this if there are bruises or broken veins.*

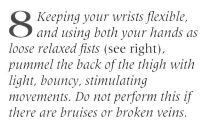

9 *Using cupped hands in a continuous, firm percussive movement (see left), massage the back of the thigh.*

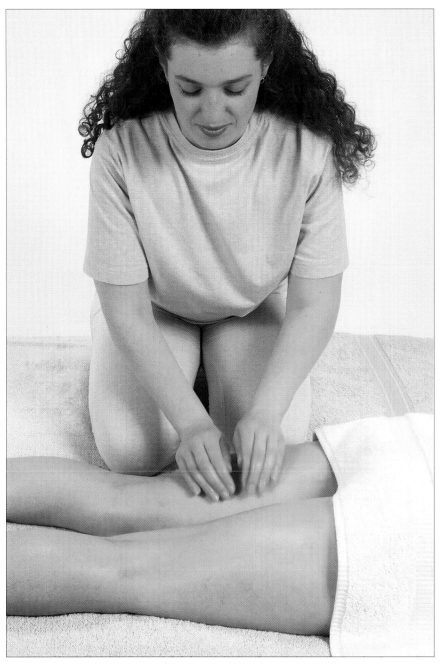

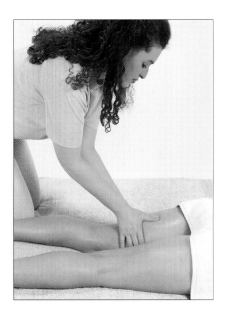

10 *The bladder meridian runs down the middle of the back of the thighs. To massage along the pathway of this meridian, position yourself as shown and use both your thumbs to press down very gently, retaining the pressure for a couple of seconds. In addition to improving circulation, this movement eases sciatica pain.*

Reposition yourself on the opposite side of the recipient, and repeat steps 1 to 10 on the other leg.

11 *Ask your partner to turn over, then cup your hands around the front of the lower leg with fingers pointing in opposite directions. Create a slight pressure by leaning in from your shoulders and use a gliding stroke up the leg, avoiding pressure on the knee. At the top of the leg, open your palms, and kneel up, leaning into the thigh. Curving your hands around the thigh, draw them down the outer leg.*

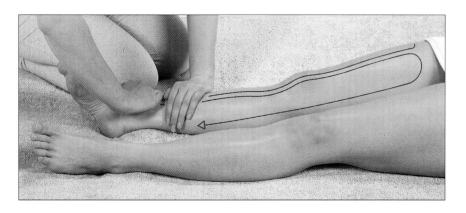

12 *Place both your hands, heels together, on the front of the thigh, with your palms and fingers wrapped around the sides. Gently lean into the heels of your hands, exerting a slight pressure from your shoulders, while sliding the heels of your hands from the centre to the outer leg. Return to the centre of the leg. Repeat the massage lower down, until you have covered the entire upper leg and thigh. Stop just before you reach the edge of the knee cap.*

13 *Place your hands side by side over the front of the thigh and, leaning into one hand, perform a petrissage wringing movement, pushing one hand over the thigh while you pull the other towards you, firmly squeezing the flesh between them.*

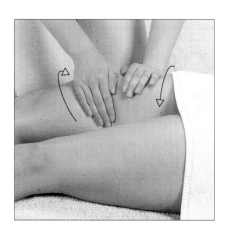

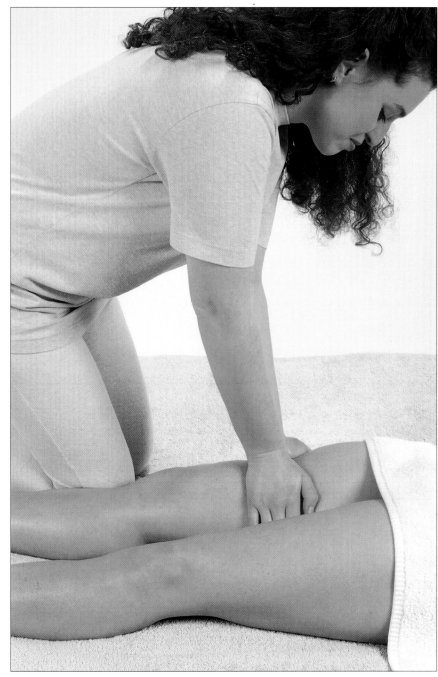

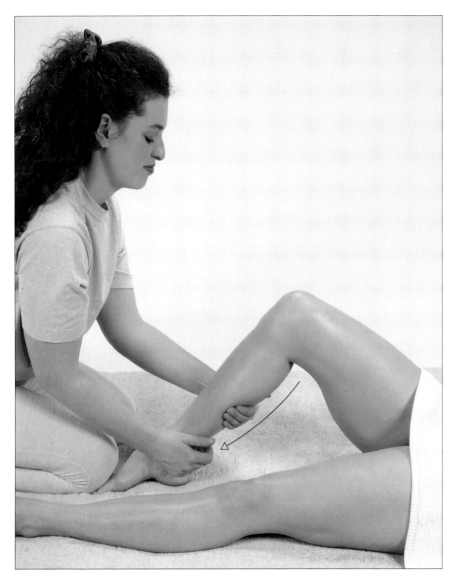

14 *Support the ankle with one hand and bend the leg resting the foot against your knees to stabilize the leg (see left). Using alternate hands, and working down towards the ankle, squeeze and release the calf muscles away from the bone, pressing the flesh between the palm of your hands and your fingers. This massage movement soothes aching legs.*

15 *Support the ankle with one hand, and, with your other hand across the bridge of the foot, gradually extend and stretch the foot by gently pulling it towards you.*

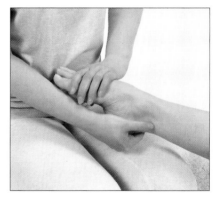

16 *Supporting the ankle (see left), place the palm of your other hand against the sole of the foot, with the heel of your hand fitting into the ball of the foot. Gently flex the foot by pushing it away from you towards the receiver's knee.*

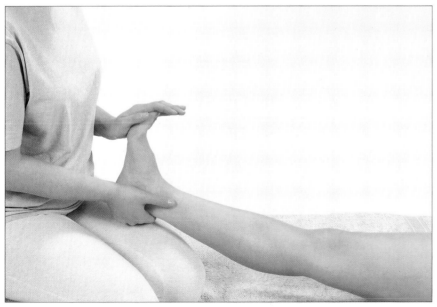

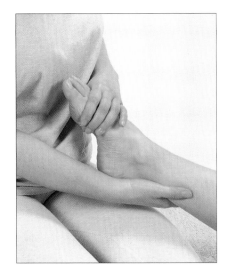

17 *Using your right hand to support the leg slightly above the ankle, hold the bridge of the toes with your left hand and gently rotate the foot from the ankle to each side. Do not force this movement, but let the foot stretch to its natural extent. Repeat twice.*

18 *Kneeling at right angles to your massage partner, support the foot and lower leg across your thighs. Hold the recipient's toes in the palm of your hand and, using your other hand with the fingers placed underneath the instep and thumb on top, rub up and down between the bones.*

19 *Support the ankle with the right hand and, using your left hand, hold the upper part of the foot. Gently pull the foot towards you and lightly shake it, vibrating the whole leg as you do so.*

Reposition yourself on the opposite side of the recipient, and repeat steps 11 to 19 on the other leg.

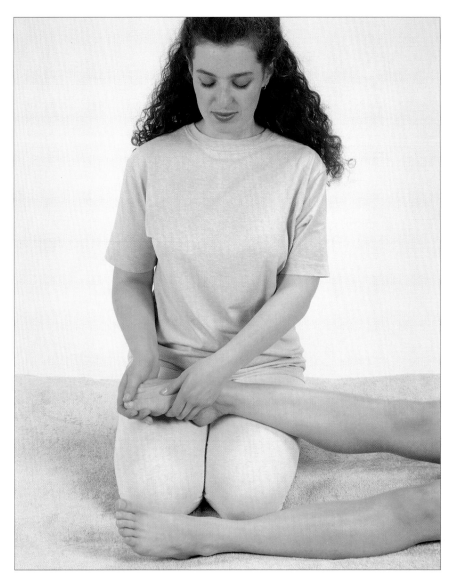

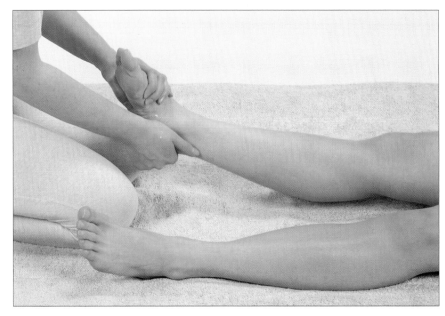

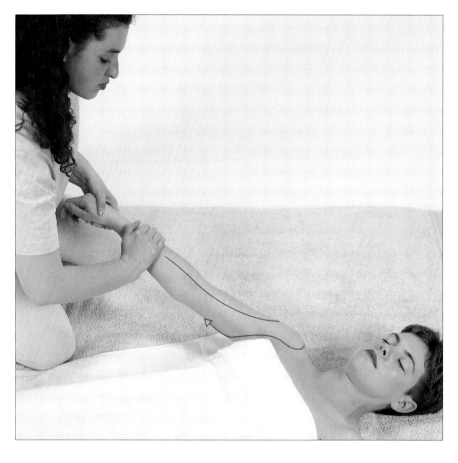

As you have completed massage techniques for the legs, first on one whole leg and foot, then on the other do the same for the arms and hands. When you have completed steps 20 to 26 on one arm and hand, reposition yourself and do them on the other.

20 *Reposition yourself, facing forwards and roughly in line with the hips of the person you are massaging (see left). Hold the wrist with one hand and cup your right hand around the arm, just above the wrist. Using the effleurage stroke, glide up the outer part of the arm to the shoulder area (see left); then glide back down the inner part of the arm, returning to the wrist. Repeat several times keeping up a steady rhythm.*

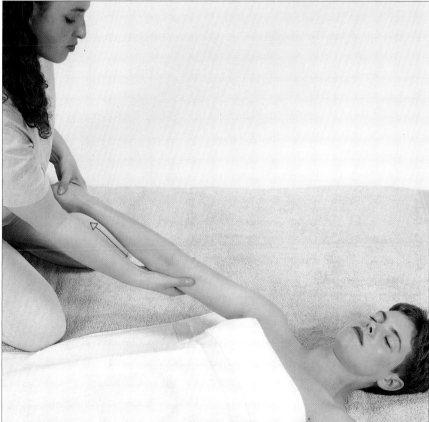

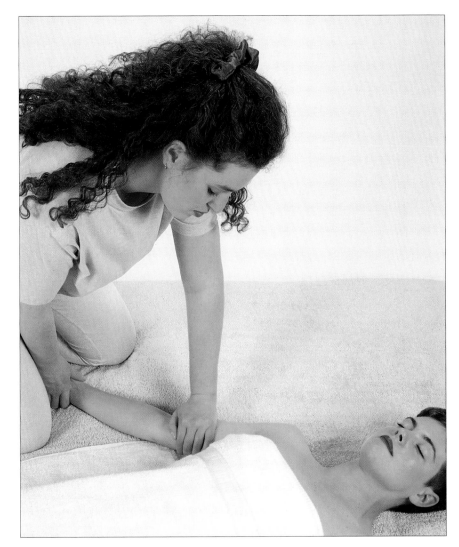

21 *With your partner's arm resting on the floor, massage gradually and rhythmically up to the shoulder area by gently squeezing and pressing down on the flesh of the arm with your palm. Kneel up so that you can lean your weight in from the shoulders. Keep your partner's arm steady by supporting it just above the wrist. Repeat a couple of times.*

22 *Sitting down on your heels once again, hold the arm up, supporting it around the wrist (see right). Using your fingers to apply moderate friction, rub up and down the arm from the wrist to shoulder area.*

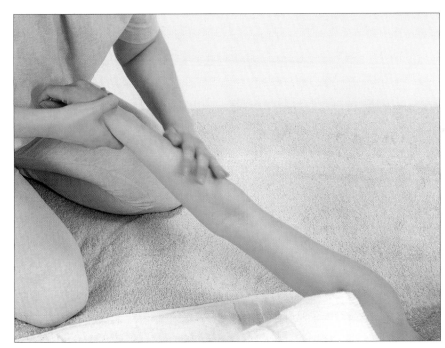

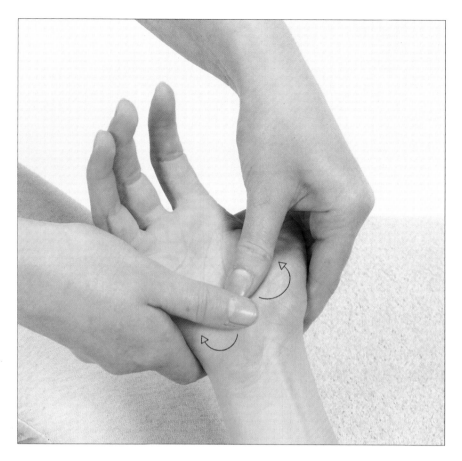

23 *Using both your hands, interlock your little fingers and ring fingers around the person's thumb and little finger (see below). Bring your other fingers underneath the hand to support and open it. Then, using your thumbs, rub with a circular pressure all over the palm area (see left).*

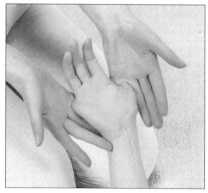

24 *With your fingers interlocked in the same position as step 23, stretch the palm by drawing the heels of your hands away from each other. Hold each stretch for a few seconds, and repeat once more.*

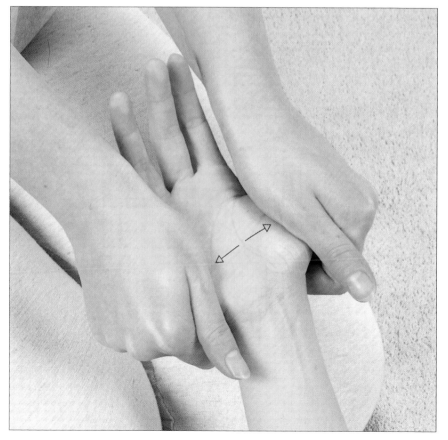

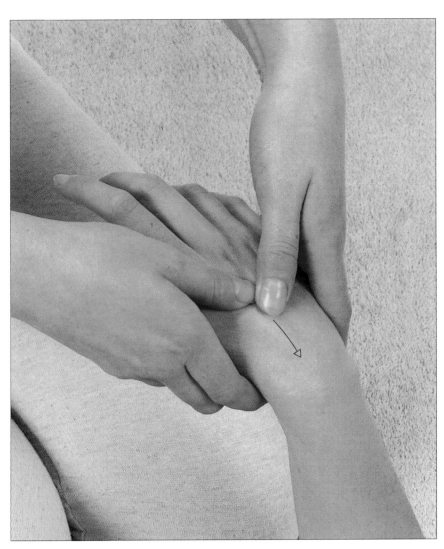

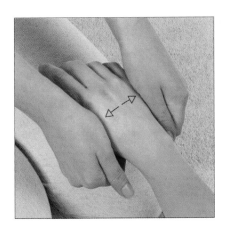

25 *Turning the hand over, clasp it on each side with the heels of your two hands meeting in the middle. Stretch the hand laterally with gentle, pulling, sliding movements, by moving the heels of your hands away from each other.*

26 *Holding the hand in the same way as for step 25, use your thumbs to stroke along the bones of the upper part of the recipient's hand, starting at the knuckles, finishing at the wrist.*

Improve Your Circulation

Nobody knows your body and its aches, pains and problem areas better than you do. This is why self-help bodywork exercises can be of such positive help when used to back up the intimate knowledge that you have about your own body and its individual – and varying – needs to be sometimes soothed, sometimes stretched, invigorated, or relaxed.

The combination of the massages given in this section, plus the self-help exercises that follow, will greatly improve poor circulation. They will help to ease the accumulation of stress and tension and any other impediments that interrupt the healthy flow of blood and lymph through the circulatory system, hindrances that can result in the kinds of health problems described on pages 53–55.

Likewise, if you are lucky enough to be problem-free and enjoying all the benefits of a good circulation, you can help yourself to retain this level of fitness, and to remain in this enviable position.

The following exercises loosen limbs, ease tensions and restrictions, increase flow of blood and nutrients, and revitalize tissues. To stimulate circulation, we can practise these exercises whenever we have had to sit for a long time, whether in an office or on an aeroplane.

1 *This exercise loosens the whole body, freeing restrictions and thus improves the circulation by enabling a beneficial flow of energy.*

Flex your torso and use both hands to rub up and down from the ankle, all over the legs, finishing at the top of the thighs. Always make sure that the rubbing includes both the front and back parts of the legs.

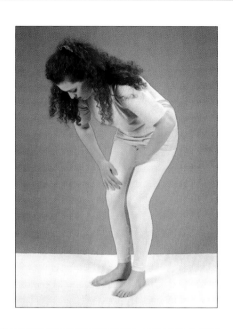

2 *This exercise helps to disperse tension and increase blood flow to the legs. It is a stimulating and re-energizing movement which helps to break up fatty deposits and congestion which impede circulation.*

Flex your torso. Keep your wrists relaxed, and make your hands into very loose and hollow fists. Work on both legs at the same time, using light bouncy pummelling movements. Begin on the outside of the legs from the buttocks to the ankles and then continue up the inside of the legs from the ankles to the thighs, being sure to include the thigh area. Repeat at least twice.

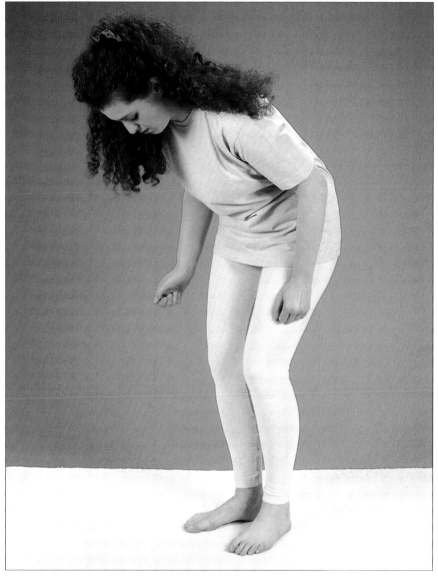

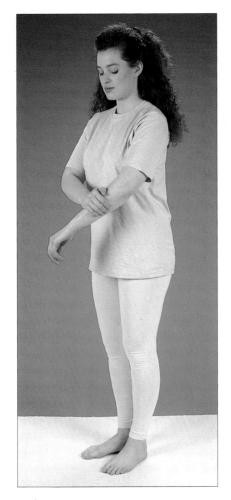

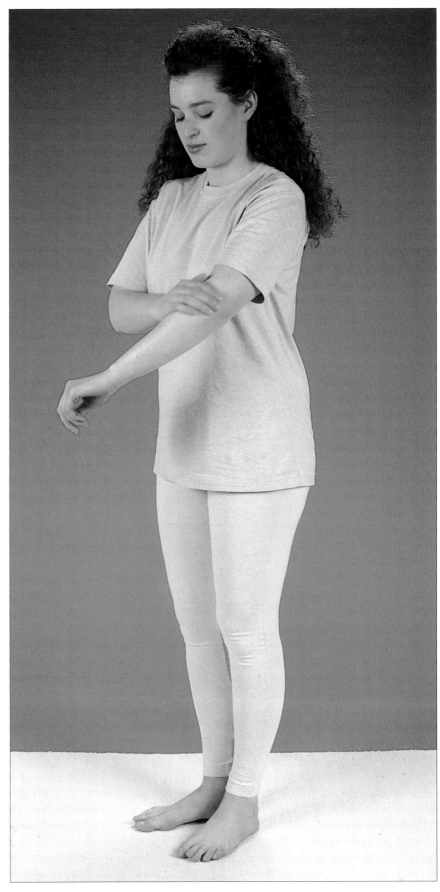

3 *This exercise, which uses a squeezing technique, releases tension and improves the flow of circulation to the arms.*

Extend your arm (see above), and, starting from your shoulder area, work all the way down to your wrist, squeezing the flesh and muscles of your arm, without pinching. Repeat on other arm.

4 *This exercise, which loosens and relaxes tense muscles, revitalizes tissues by bringing a fresh supply of blood and nutrients.*

Keeping your arm extended, rub vigorously up and down the entire length of your arm, starting from your wrist. Repeat on other arm.

CHAPTER THREE

Flexible Joints

It is astonishing how many moving parts our bodies have, and not surprising that the joints that are most vulnerable to wear and tear and loss of flexibility are those that we use the most: spine, neck, elbows, hands, wrists, hips and knees. The decrease in flexibility as we grow older can result in inflammation – arthritis – in the joints, and other problems. We can help our joints to remain mobile, however.

The Structure of Joints

The human body has more than two hundred joints, each designed to allow varying degrees of movement; and to reduce the wear and tear and loss of mobility, the friction between the surfaces has to be kept to a minimum.

Fixed joints (immovable)
Some joints, for example the joints between the individual bones of the skull, are classified as fixed or immovable, however, some osteopaths believe there is some imperceptible movement.

Semi-joints (slightly movable)
The second type of joints are described as semi- or slightly movable, as between the vertebrae or individual bones of the pelvis. Between these bones there are discs and movement is only possible by compressing these tough pad-like structures *(see Chapter One, Spinal Structures page 28)*.

Freely-movable joints
The third type are called freely-movable joints and these, as the term suggests, allow the greatest degree of movement possible in a specific area. These comprise mostly the joints of the limbs and extremities, such as the shoulder, elbow, hip, knee and ankle. Freely-movable joints have some characteristics in common:

Cartilage. This connective tissue covers the parts of bone that form the joint, and is found in joints such as the shoulder and knee, allowing the joints to move without friction.

Capsule. This membraneous sac, which encloses and protects joints and keeps bones connected, is similar to a ligament, and is commonly referred to as capsular ligament.

Synovial membrane. Sited beneath the capsule is this membrane which secretes synovial fluid. This acts mainly as a lubricant for the various structures of the joint.

Joints, then, are enclosed in a capsule, lined with synovial membrane, lubricated by synovial fluid, and externally strengthened (or held together) by ligaments. To allow for a variety of movements, joints function in different ways *(see Bones and Joints, page 70)*.

Common Complaints

Any inflammatory or degenerative condition that affects joints is termed arthritis. Massage and bodywork, acupressure, diet, essential oils and herbal teas help to avoid or alleviate the pain of this and other joint problems, from frozen shoulder to water on the knee.

Osteoarthritis
This common wear-and-tear complaint mainly affects larger joints in older people. Weight-bearing structures, such as the hip, weaken, resulting in degenerative changes and over-stress that damage the joint surfaces and produce pain and disability. Causes can be poor posture, obesity, and injuries, such as a heavy fall and fractures.

The disease starts in the cartilage, which

BONES AND JOINTS

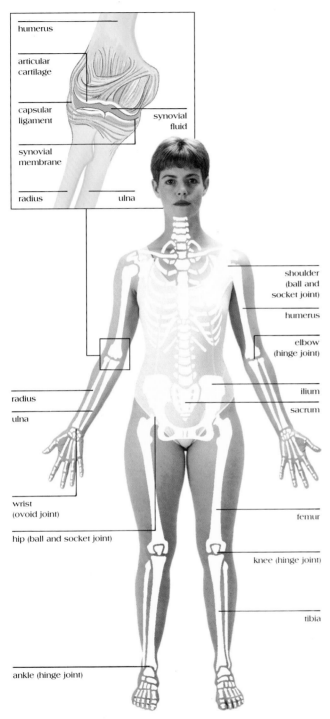

humerus

articular cartilage

capsular ligament

synovial fluid

synovial membrane

radius   ulna

shoulder (ball and socket joint)

humerus

elbow (hinge joint)

ilium

sacrum

radius

ulna

wrist (ovoid joint)

femur

hip (ball and socket joint)

knee (hinge joint)

tibia

ankle (hinge joint)

The elbow, ankle and knee have hinge joints, the wrist has an ovoid (egg-shaped) joint. The shoulder and hip ball-and-socket joints while the first two cervical vertebrae have pivot joints. The movement of these joints is assisted by cartilage, and synovial membrane, which secretes synovial fluid (see inset).

begins to thin out and no longer protects the bones forming the joint. The pain is worse when standing and moving, and the resulting symptoms, such as inflammation, swelling and heat, severely limit movement and can cause surrounding muscles to waste due to inactivity.

Massage and bodywork brings some relief by helping to ease the pain of muscles that surround the joints; by improving circulation to the area; and by gently stretching the joints and possibly reducing friction between bone surfaces. *(For massage and bodywork concerning particular joints, see the relevant chapters, such as Chapter One, page 28, for vertebral joints; and Chapter Eight, page 113, for the neck.)*

Rheumatoid arthritis

This occurs more often in women than in men. It tends to affect the connective tissues, in particular, the areas around and within smaller peripheral joints, such as the hands and feet. Because connective tissue keeps many structures connected to each other, rheumatoid arthritis can be widespread throughout the body.

It is characterized by pain, severe inflammation around the affected joint or joints, and hardening of synovial membranes. When advanced, there is progressive fusing of joints or partial dislocations, and the joint becomes swollen and very restricted in movement. This can result in severe muscle-wasting, and visible deformity. The person feels feverish, fatigued, weak and generally unwell and depressed.

The exact cause is still unknown, but indications point to the influence of infection or toxaemia – a build up of toxins which create inflammation and degeneration and trigger self-destructive immune responses. Antibodies reach the site of inflammation to combat the infection only to worsen the condition. If it involves just one joint, it is possible to contain or slow down the progression of the illness.

If tackled in the early stages, massage, using the essential oils *(see page 75)* or cream *(see page 74)*, is very beneficial for improving this condition. To begin with, the massage should be very mild and gradual, just gently massaging around

A HEALTHY DIET FOR RHEUMATOID ARTHRITIS

Diet is considered of paramount importance for this condition, and the following foods should be avoided while treating rheumatism with natural methods: red meat; pork and all its derivatives, such as ham, bacon; deep-fried food, such as fish and chips; sugar and everything that contains it, such as cakes and soft drinks. Consume alcohol, tomatoes and citrus fruits only in moderation.

HERBAL REMEDIES FOR RHEUMATOID ARTHRITIS

Between meals, drink one or two cups a day of the following herbal mixture: corn silk *(Zea mays)*, dandelion root or herb *(Taraxacum officinale)*, heartsease *(Viola tricolor)*, plantain herb *(Plantago officinalis)*.

Mix the herbs well and infuse 5 mg (1 teaspoon) in a cup of hot water for ten minutes. Strain the herbs before drinking.

You can also purchase the same mixture in tincture form. In this instance, add ten-to-fifteen drops to a glass of water. If you are using the tincture, ask your herbalist to add devil's claw *(Harpagophytum procumbens)* to the mixture.

If you are not including devil's claw in your herbal tea, you can purchase it in tablet form from a health food store; take two tablets a day.

all the affected areas. Later on, the therapist can slowly and gently mobilize the restricted joints.

For acupressure treatment, rub the following points using a circular motion for two minutes, three times a week: SP 6 *(see Chapter Two, page 55)*, CO 11, LIV 3 and KID 3 *(see page 72)*.

Frozen shoulder

This common and painful condition of the shoulder affects the muscles, tendons and joint structures. It usually begins with inflammation of the tendons that move the shoulder, or of the fibrous capsule or joint, or swelling of the sac that cushions the joint. Limited movement ranges from mild to severe.

The pain at its most severe can make movement impossible. It is worsened by shoulder movements, such as combing or brushing hair.

Massage, often as a supplement to other therapies like physiotherapy, certainly can help. Having massaged and warmed the muscles around the shoulder and the upper back area, the articulatory techniques described here for the shoulder will help to mobilize the area. Start the techniques very slowly and constantly monitor the person you are articulating for any sign of pain or discomfort. This condition gradually responds to regular treatment, and osteopathic manipulation can help hasten recovery and restore movement. Also helpful are hot baths to which you have added five to seven drops of the essential oils of lavender or chamomile.

Repetitive stress injury (RSI)

This term applies to any painful injury and inflammation in the body, limbs and extremities caused by repetitive movements, such as repeatedly pulling on the same muscles, for example, while working at a computer, gardening, or sports. It is made worse by poor posture.

Massage, as a supplement to physiotherapy, helps dispel stiffness, tension and pain in the affected joint. First concentrate the massage on the afflicted area – such as fingers, wrists, elbow or neck.

Having said that, the neck and shoulder massage sequences in this book are beneficial for helping to counteract and reduce muscle fatigue and strain, such common features of RSI.

For acupressure treatment, massage the following points for five minutes each day: PE 6 *(see Chapter Two, page 55)* for pain and cramp, and CO 4 *(see page 72)* for pain in the hand.

Tennis elbow

The hinged joint of the elbow is particularly vulnerable to injury, sprains and dislocations. The condition is caused by frequent minor jarring of the joint (as in tennis, from which it takes its name, or in everyday activities, such as typing or hammering). It involves strain of the muscles and tendons on the outer side of the elbow joint. The result is pain and stiffness.

Resting the elbow by avoiding the action that has caused the condition is the first step. Then massage, using gentle effleurage and petrissage kneadings, will relieve the pain.

When the acute discomfort has passed, deeper finger friction and kneading of the muscles surrounding the elbow will further help recovery. Gentle manipulation of the joint, by an osteopath, will also help to restore mobility. For acupressure treatment, massage CO 11 *(see below)* for two minutes each day.

ACUPRESSURE POINTS

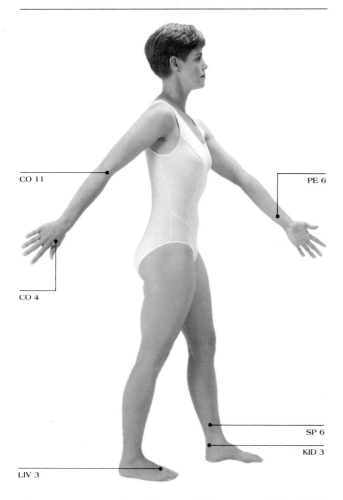

CO 11

PE 6

CO 4

SP 6

KID 3

LIV 3

The acupressure points illustrated above are all beneficial for easing and soothing joint problems, thus helping restore movement. PE 6 and CO 4 are especially useful for repetitive stress injury; CO 11 can alleviate tennis elbow; LIV 3, SP 6, CO 4 and KID 3 all help rheumatoid arthritis. Massage the appropriate points with a circular pressure for two minutes as required.

Synovitis (water on the knee)
The synovial membrane secretes fluid to lubricate joints, but when there is injury an excess of this fluid is secreted in an attempt to heal. Before trying any treatment, the presence of a major lesion must always be eliminated. In many cases minor injuries, which have caused no damage to the knee, are followed by a persistent accumulation of fluid. Massage with essential oils, using the strokes shown here, will help to reduce this excess fluid problem, and ease the inflammation. *(See the massage and self-help techniques for circulation on pages 51–68).*

Acupressure Points

Use PE 6 *(page 55)* and CO 4 for repetitive stress injury; CO 11 for tennis elbow; LIV 3, SP 6 *(page 55)*, CO 4 and KID 3 for rheumatoid arthritis.

Colon 4 (CO 4). Located on the fleshy part of the back of the hand between the thumb and the index finger. Because the colon meridian from the hand reaches the face, this point relieves pain and inflammation in the face, and also of colds. CO 4 is also used for intestinal problems such as constipation and irritable bowel syndrome. Also a good point to relieve sudden weakness, shock, fainting, hand pain and arthritis. Do not use during pregnancy, or in conjunction with SP 6, if the receiver complains of excessive menstrual flow.

Colon 11 (CO 11). When the elbow is flexed, this point is located at the end of the crease on the outer bone of the arm. This is a good point for local pain in the elbow. It also removes heat and toxicity from the blood, therefore helping in skin conditions like acne and intestinal problems like diarrhoea and colitis.

Liver 3 (LIV 3). In the flesh close to where the bones of the big and second toes meet. This point helps to clear the liver. It can be used for soreness in the right upper side of the abdomen, bitter taste in the mouth, biliousness and liverish headaches.

Kidney 3 (KID 3). Go to the tip of the inner ankle bone; the point is one cun away in a straight parallel line towards the Achilles' tendon.

Shoulder, Knee and Pelvic Massage

You will find many massage, bodywork and self-help techniques throughout this book that help to stretch and release joints that have become painful and immobile. See, for example, articulations to stretch the back *(Chapter One)*; techniques to stretch ankle and foot, wrist and hand *(Chapter Two)*, and the neck *(Chapter Eight)*. In addition to techniques in other chapters, the following massages will help to keep healthy joints flexible.

Massage and bodywork can do much to help prevent distressing problems with the joints from occurring in the first place. Exercise and a healthy diet make a great contribution to maintaining flexible joints.

When a condition already exists, these massages will help you to avoid or ease the pain that arises when areas around them become inflamed and swollen, and the joints themselves are stiff and restricted. To perform the techniques, first kneel down alongside your massage partner's chest.

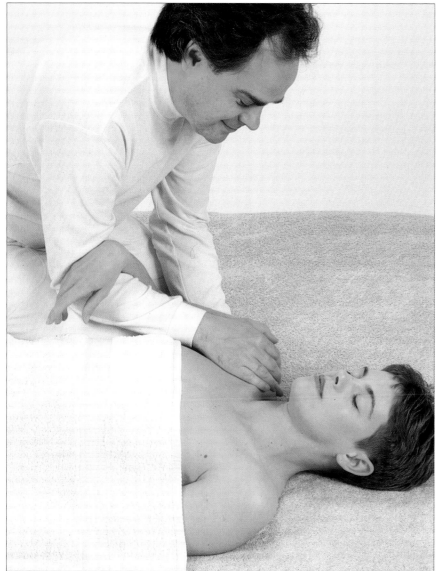

1 *Place your left hand beneath the right shoulder joint and your right hand on top of the shoulder. The right wrist should rest comfortably over your right elbow. Then, with both your hands moving together, slowly rotate the shoulder joint in a circle. Repeat a few times.*

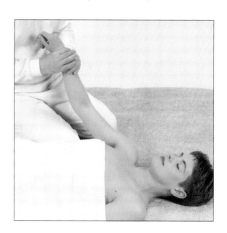

2 *Raise the arm using both your hands, hold the wrist securely, then gently pull and shake the arm up and down (see above) so that the shoulder joint feels as if it is being gently extended – stretched.*

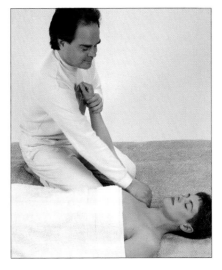

3 *Hold the receiver's right wrist and hand with your left hand. Using only the palm and heel of your right hand, gently squeeze the muscles of the shoulder, working all over the area.*

As a variation for this exercise, use your left hand to gently pull the arm towards you and with your right hand, press against the shoulder joint in an upward movement for a few seconds. Repeat twice.

4 *Place the receiver's arm across their chest with the right hand on the left shoulder. Place your left hand on their right shoulder and your right hand on their right elbow. Gently and slowly push from the shoulder toward the elbow for a few seconds until you feel the shoulder extending, stretching. Repeat twice.*

Reposition yourself and repeat steps 1 to 4 on the other shoulder.

MASSAGE CREAM FOR RHEUMATOID ARTHRITIS

To 65 g (2½ oz) aqueous cream, add the following essential oils: three drops of lavender, two of juniper and two of chamomile. Then add 15 ml (1 tablespoon) of each of the following tinctures: marsh mallow root *(Althaea officinalis)*, plantain *(Plantago officinalis)*, burdock root *(Arctium lappa)*, and ash leaves *(Fraxinus excelsior)*.

Mix well and, to soothe joint pain and inflammation, use a small amount for massage twice a day.

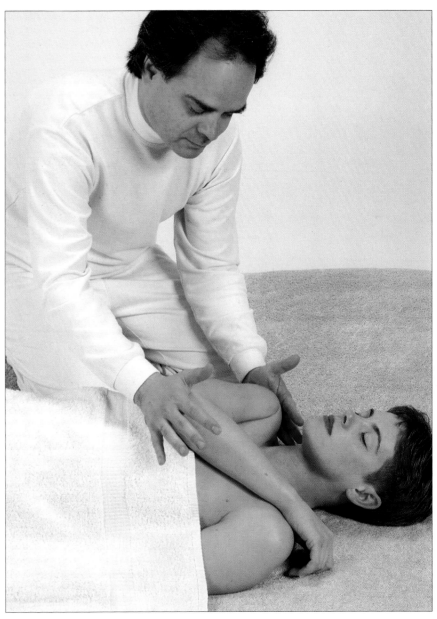

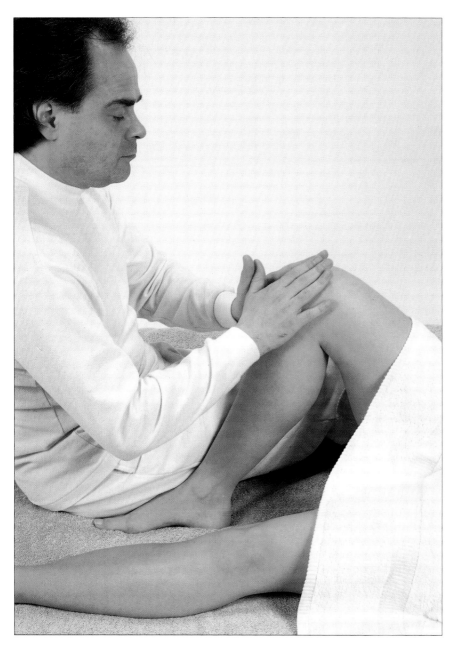

MASSAGE OILS FOR JOINT PROBLEMS

Add the following essential oils to 30 ml (2 tablespoons) of base oil.

Osteoarthritis: two drops each of lavender and chamomile.

Rheumatoid arthritis: two drops of lavender and one drop of juniper.

Frozen shoulder: two drops each of lavender and chamomile, or juniper and rosemary.

Synovitis (water on the knee): two drops each of juniper and lavender.

Tennis elbow: two drops each of lavender and chamomile.

When you have completed steps 5 to 7 reposition yourself and repeat these steps on the other leg. Then ask your partner to turn over for steps 8 and 9 working on the sacro-iliac joint.

5 *Move, so that you are sitting alongside your partner's lower leg. Bend their leg at the knee and rest the foot under your thigh to stabilize the leg. Then, with your hands moving in opposite directions, massage by rubbing in circular movements around the entire knee.*

6 *Keeping the foot resting against your thigh to stabilize the leg, use the heels of your hands to massage the knee joint with gentle, but firm circular movements on both sides of the knee (see left).*

7 *In the same position with your fingers behind the knee, place your thumbs on the gaps either side of the knee joint. This is where the thigh bone (femur) meets the bone of the lower leg (tibia). Make moderate circular rubbing pressures all round this area for 3 or 4 minutes.*

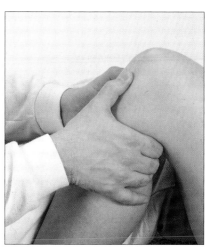

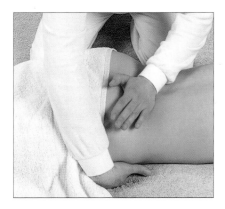

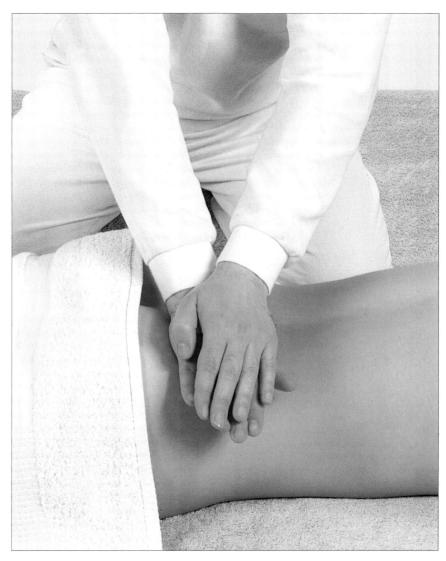

8 *Kneeling opposite the receiver's pelvis and leaning across their back, place your right hand beneath the right pelvic bone (ilium), and your left hand on the edge of the upper part of the pelvic bone. You will find this just above the right dimple of the lower back, above the buttocks. Now gently rock the pelvic bone back and forwards so that you create a slight gap between the joint of the pelvic bone and the sacrum.*

9 *Place one hand on top of the other on the edges of the pelvic bone that run from the sacrum to the waist. Working from that point, using the heel of your hand, rub and stretch the muscles in an outward or side-to-side movement. Repeat steps 8 and 9 on other side.*

Self-help for Flexible Joints

The following exercises can be used both for keeping joints in good condition, and for gently easing and releasing joints which have become stiff, inflexible and painful. These effects could be due to inflammatory conditions, such as arthritis, or other problems, such as frozen shoulder, repetitive stress injury, tennis elbow and water on the knee, caused by straining or over-using the muscles and ligaments around joints and the tendons on each side of them.

If movement has become severely limited and restricted, it will take time and regular practice sessions before flexibility is restored.

Be gentle with yourself, and do not repeat any exercises that cause you more pain. It is also inadvisable to exercise when joint problems are at the acute stage and any kind of movement worsens the pain. At times such as these, rub the affected area with cream *(see page 74)* or relax in bath water to which you have added essential oils *(see page 75)*. You will know the right moment to begin helping to restore a joint's mobility by using the self-help exercises on a regular basis – and the other appropriate exercises included throughout this book.

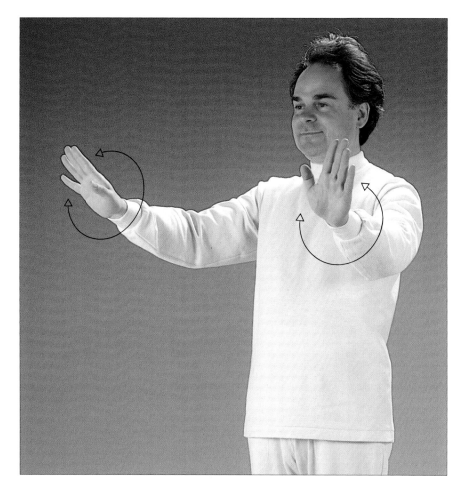

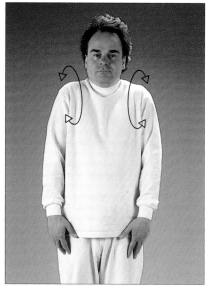

1 *You can stand or sit to do this. Hold your torso straight, but not tensed, and slowly raise and rotate your shoulders a few times, first in one direction, then the other.*

2 *Hold your arms out straight and, keeping your hands relaxed, rotate the wrists a few times first in one direction, then the other.*

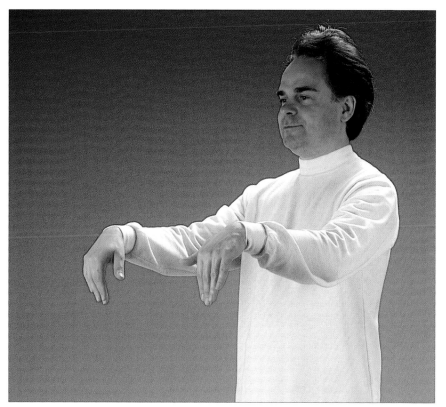

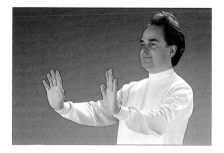

3 *Holding your arms out straight, with your hands relaxed (as in step 2), flex and extend your wrists by bringing your hands up as far as they will go (see above) and then down (left). Repeat this a few times ensuring that you are bending from the wrists not from the fingers.*

4 *Slightly bend your body, including your knees, and place both your hands over your knees (see right). Then, keeping your hands relaxed on your knees, rotate your knees a few times, moving them first in one direction, then the other.*

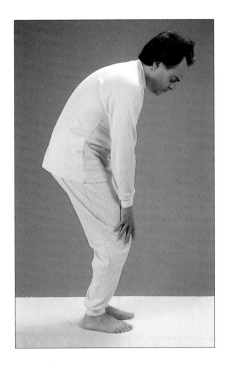

5 *Maintain the same relaxed slightly bent position as in step 4, keeping both your hands placed on your knees. Then extend and flex your knees by a series of actions in which you move your knees back and forth, straightening your legs as you do so. Repeat this a few times.*

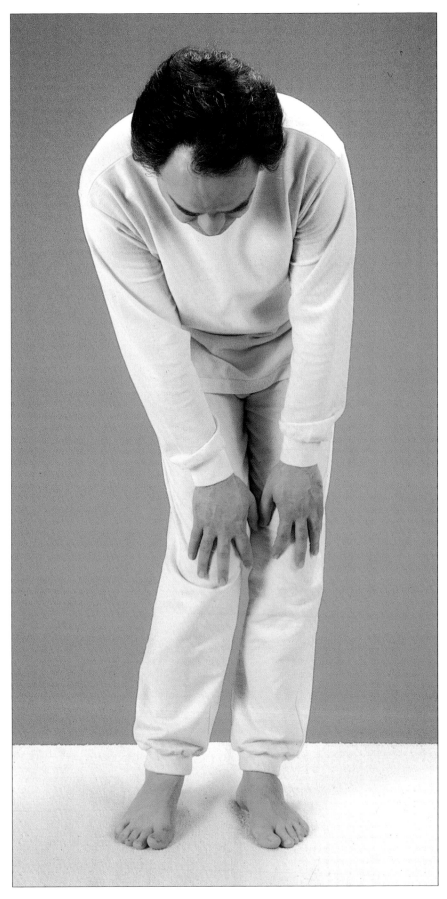

CHAPTER FOUR
Better Breathing

The respiratory system brings to us the one most important substance that each cell requires – oxygen. If illness or musculo-skeletal abnormalities prevent our bodies from taking in an adequate amount, we cannot thrive. However, the respiratory system is often impaired by various infections and pollutants and needs to be strengthened regularly by therapeutic approaches like massage and breathing exercises. Through use of the appropriate techniques we can free the rib cage and chest, thus improving respiration and immunity.

The Respiratory System

Through the respiratory system oxygen is taken into the body and carbon dioxide, a waste product from cell metabolism, is excreted. Its main organ is the two lungs but it also comprises the nose, the pharynx (throat), the larynx (voice box), the trachea, the bronchi, the covering of the lungs called the pleura and the respiration muscles: intercostal muscles and diaphragm.

Therefore respiratory complaints not only affect the lungs, but also involve areas like the nose, sinuses, eustachian tubes, ears and throat. A problem like an ear infection can be relieved by treating points along the lung meridian, and by using essential oils that help to clear infections in the respiratory system.

The first important consideration for a massage therapist is that respiration depends greatly on the intercostal muscles and the diaphragm. The diaphragm divides the chest from the abdomen, while the intercostal muscles cover all the mid portion of the torso attaching it to the lower ribs, sternum and vertebral column. During inspiration the ribs and intercostal muscles expand; the diaphragm

THE RIB CAGE

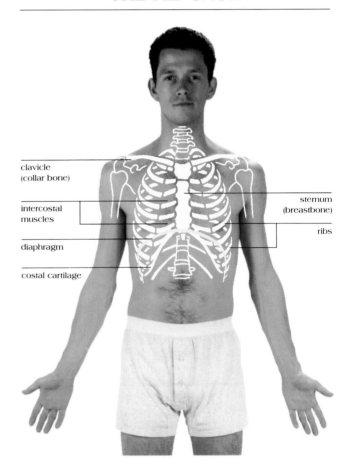

clavicle (collar bone)

intercostal muscles

diaphragm

costal cartilage

sternum (breastbone)

ribs

The curved rib bones form a protective cage around the heart, lungs and other internal organs, and are a framework for the chest. There are twelve pairs of ribs, each pair joined at the back of the rib cage to a vertebra in the spine. Covering the ribs is intercostal muscle, which, with the diaphragm, expands the chest.

descends allowing the lungs to stretch and inflate with oxygen. During expiration these muscles contract forcing the ribs in and the diaphragm ascends pushing air out of the lungs. The diaphragm can be constricted by many

79

factors, one being digestion. If the abdomen is congested and swollen by retention of food, it can obstruct the descent of the diaphragm during inspiration which creates shallow breathing.

So, muscular, rib and vertebral restrictions, and tension can severely impair the respiratory system. If the lungs cannot properly expand to take in oxygen or fully eliminate carbon dioxide, the body may gradually feel weaker and more intoxicated and we also become more prone to respiratory infections. Massage and bodywork can relax the muscles, open the ribs and stretch the thoracic vertebrae. This will strengthen the respiratory system and increase our immunity and general vitality.

The second major consideration of a massage therapist is that breathing, particularly the muscular contraction and relaxation, is also controlled by centres in the brain stem. Therefore prolonged nervous and emotional tension can easily contract unduly the muscles of respiration and contribute to poor respiration. Again massage is very effective in promoting relaxation; when we are relaxed and at peace our breathing becomes deeper and more regular.

Using massage to work on areas like the head and below the occiput (base of the head), where the vagus nerve emerges, can contribute greatly to relaxation and better breathing.

If you are prone to chest complaints and you live in a city, you need to regenerate your lungs in a cleaner atmosphere. Take frequent trips to the fresh air of the countryside, the mountains or the sea. If you are a smoker try to cut it to a minimum. An exercise regime, tailored to your needs and capacity, is also recommended.

Lastly, remember that, according to all the schools of natural medicine, diet plays an important role in maintaining the health of your lungs. In my practical experience I have found it to be true, particularly for those suffering from accumulation of mucus in the respiratory area with associated conditions such as coughs, bronchial asthma and bronchitis. A diet rich in fats, such as deep fried foods or dairy products gives rise to over production of mucus.

THE RESPIRATORY SYSTEM

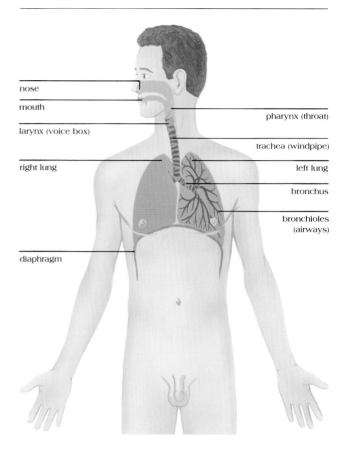

nose
mouth
larynx (voice box)
right lung
diaphragm

pharynx (throat)
trachea (windpipe)
left lung
bronchus
bronchioles (airways)

In addition to the lungs, the respiratory system comprises various respiratory passages. The nose or the mouth are the pathways by which air containing oxygen enters and leaves the body as we breathe. Via the pharynx, then the trachea and bronchus the air is pulled into the lungs by the intercostal muscles and diaphragm.

This mucus obstructs the respiratory passages.

The techniques shown in this chapter can be further enhanced by other massage techniques such as the ones that relax the upper back and the shoulders. (*See particularly techniques on pages 46–7 of Chapter One and those included in Chapter Eight, pages 117–25 and 129–37.*)

Common Complaints

Massage, with its strengthening and soothing benefits, can often contribute to preventing some of the most common respiratory complaints, such as colds or flu and mucus

problems. Massage can also enable our bodies to cope with them better when they do occur.

Colds and flu

The common cold is a viral infection causing inflammation of the mucous membranes lining the nose and throat, resulting in a runny nose, possibly headache and sore throat. Flu or influenza, also a viral infection of the respiratory system, brings fever, aching of both the head and muscles and weakness. There is no known cure. Antibiotics are prescribed at times to lessen the side effects of a flu affecting the bronchi and the ears.

Massage, essential oils and herbs can help reduce the severity of the symptoms and shorten the duration of the infection. *(See Herbal Tea for Colds and Flu below.)*

Also reputed to be of benefit in fighting a cold are vitamin C, found in citrus fruits and leafy vegetables, and zinc, a trace element found in lean meat, wholemeal breads and seafood. Ask your health food shop to advise you on other sources of vitamin C and zinc.

For massage, add one or two of the following essential oils to a saucer of 30 ml (2 tablespoons) of base oil, either two drops of one oil or one drop each of two oils: peppermint, eucalyptus, benzoin. Massage the combination over the chest, forehead, neck and upper back.

For colds and flu, you can also massage the following acupressure points: BL 12 *(see Chapter One, page 33)*; CO 4 *(see Chapter Three, page 72)*; LU 1 and LU 5 *(see page 83)*.

HERBAL TEA FOR COLDS AND FLU

At the onset of symptoms make yourself a cup of herbal tea, 5 mg (1 teaspoon) infused in a cup of hot water for ten minutes of the following herbs mixed in equal parts: bonset *(Eupatorium perfoliatum)*, elder flowers *(Sambucus nigra)* and peppermint leaves *(Mentha piperita)*. Strain and drink it while warm and have three cups a day. Particularly have a cup before retiring at night and try to induce sweating by keeping well covered. For dosing children refer to page 18.

TREATMENT FOR HAY FEVER AND ALLERGIES

Massage the upper body areas such as the neck, upper back, chest and head *(see pages 34–43 and 117–32)*, using essential oils such as lavender, eucalyptus and benzoin. Also massage the lung meridian especially points in it like LU 1 and LU 5 *(see page 83)*. Use gentle and calming techniques around the nose and eyes. Freeing the neck can also help to drain mucus and lymph from the head, thus helping to relieve and prevent some of the symptoms of hay fever.

Hay fever and allergies

Hay fever (allergic rhinitis) is an abnormal immune reaction to pollens, plants or dust. It occurs from spring to late summer, depending on area and types of pollens. There is irritation of the mucous membranes of the nose and upper respiratory tract; perhaps nasal discharge and obstruction, oedema around the eyes with excessive and painful lacrimation, sneezing, coughing and difficult breathing. For some the symptoms are mild, but for others they can be quite extreme. People allergic to dust may have less severe reactions, but are exposed year round.

In most cases, bodywork and natural therapies might not offer a cure, but they may lessen and prevent some of the most difficult symptoms. Also, a few weeks before the expected onset of symptoms, avoid an excessive intake of mucus-producing and irritating foods like dairy products, sugar and cakes, white bread, fried food, hot and spicy food and alcohol.

'Weak lungs'

This condition, also referred to as 'weak immunity', may not be in most Western medical books, but natural and traditional medicine places great importance on the relationship between the lungs and immunity. When people complain of continuously catching colds, flus and other respiratory infections, they have weak immunity. They are also tired, and possibly emaciated.

The massage techniques can go a long away in strengthening the lungs of these individuals

HERBAL TREATMENT FOR 'WEAK LUNGS'

I would advise the following herbal tea for anyone suffering from 'weak lungs'. Drink one cup of tea a day, 5 mg (1 teaspoon) infused for ten minutes in a cup of hot water, of the following mixture in equal parts: plantain (*Plantago officinalis*), borage (*Borago officinalis*) and mullein (*Verbascum thapsus*). The same advice given for 'weak lungs' is also valid for emphysema, a disease in which the alveoli (tiny air sacs) in the lungs become damaged.

HERBAL TEA FOR MUCUS PROBLEMS

Mix the following in equal parts: violet leaves (*Viola odorata*), coltsfoot leaves (*Tussilago farfara*) (avoid during pregnancy), peppermint leaves (*Mentha piperita*) and mullein flowers (*Verbascum thapsus*). Infuse 5 mg (1 teaspoon) of the mixture for ten minutes in a cup of hot water. Drink two cups a day at least one hour before or after meals. Can be purchased in tincture form; have fifteen drops in a cup of warm water twice a day. For dosing children refer to page 18.

particularly if they follow the exercises under the section on self-help *(see page 87)*.

During the massage you can use essential oils like eucalyptus, frankincense or benzoin.

Mucus problems

This heading covers conditions like sinusitis, bronchitis, cough with expectoration and bronchial asthma, described below. *(See Herbal Tea for Mucus Problems.)*

The lungs are in constant contact with air therefore many kinds of pollutants are carried into them. The membranes that cover the upper part of the respiratory system like the nose and the bronchi should give protection. They exude moderate amounts of mucus to trap pollutants, allergens (like pollen and car fumes) and bacteria. When this mucus is expectorated the trapped pollutants are safely thrown off the respiratory system. During various infections or allergic irritations the membranes can be severely irritated; an excessive production of mucus then gets trapped in areas of the respiratory system such as the sinuses, the nose, the throat and the bronchi.

Sinusitis. An infection leads to inflammation of the membrane lining the facial sinuses, the air-filled cavities in the bone around the nose. There is a feeling of fullness, perhaps a throbbing ache, and excess mucus drains into the nasal cavity. Usually affected are the maxillary sinuses in the cheekbones, and the ethmoidal sinuses between the eyes. *(See Herbal Tea; see also Chapter Eight, step 5, page 130.)*

Cough with Expectoration. Phlegm (sputum) is produced due to irritation of the upper respiratory tract, often in seemingly large quantities, which causes discomfort and perhaps breathing problems. Massage can help to 'loosen' a cough, by stimulating expectoration of mucus from the lungs.

Bronchitis. The bronchi, the airways that connect the trachea (windpipe) to the lungs, become inflamed due to viral infection. A cough results, often producing large quantities of phlegm. Both acute bronchitis (sudden, of short duration) and the chronic form (persistent over time) are more common among smokers and those who live in areas of high pollution.

Bronchial asthma. This condition is caused by obstruction of the bronchial airways. Mucus is accompanied by spasmodic constriction, inflammation and swelling in the bronchial area. The symptoms can be distressing. There may be difficulty in breathing, wheezing and accompanying anxiety.

Mucus problems can be relieved through the use of massage and natural treatments. These aim to strengthen the respiratory system by opening the musculo-skeletal system that controls it; they also help to eliminate bacterial infections, and to strengthen the expectorant capacity of the lungs.

In addition to the techniques illustrated in this chapter, you can use some of those for the upper back, neck and face, particularly the techniques on pages 128–32. Remember also to try to follow the sound dietary advice given

throughout the introductory part of this chapter.

Essential oils can be very effective in helping any of these mucus problems. In a saucer of 30 ml (2 tablespoons) of base oil, add two drops of one essential oil or one drop each of two chosen essential oils. Those recommended are: eucalyptus, benzoin, fennel, frankincense, mandarin.

Acupressure Points

Use of the following acupressure points can help to relieve some respiratory complaints and strengthen the respiratory system.

Lung 1 (LU 1). Located one cun below the outside edge of the collar bone (clavicle) or highest point of the collar bone near to the shoulder. Used for fullness and tightness of the lungs, asthma, coughs and mucus problems.

Lung 5 (LU 5). Found on the elbow crease close to the outer and slightly shorter of the two forearm bones which extend from the elbow to the wrist and next to the outside edge of the biceps muscles tendon. This tendon can be felt easily when you tense the arm. Good point for chronic ailments of the lungs, particularly if due to mucus retention. LU 5 is also used to help allay chronic colds.

BL 12 and CO 4 are also useful acupressure points for the relief of respiratory problems. A description of how to locate BL 12 is given in Chapter One *(see page 33)* and of CO 4 in Chapter Three *(see page 72)*.

ACUPRESSURE POINTS

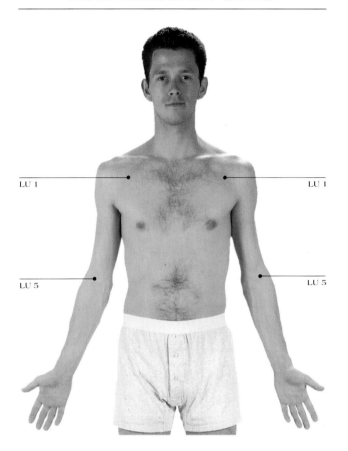

The acupressure points are important to the therapist and to the receiver. Tapping these channels of internal energy flow are a positive way to encourage the respiratory system to function fully. The points to aid breathing, shown above, help both to clear the respiratory system of mucus and increase respiratory capacity.

Massage for Better Breathing

For those of us lucky enough to have a healthy respiratory system, it is essential to maintain it. Massage can help to do so. For those who suffer from respiratory complaints, massage can bring strength and resilience as well as comfort and pleasure.

Remember that a healthy diet is an important starting point for improvement to any area of the body *(see page 80)*. Then, follow the breathing exercises recommended in this chapter *(see page 87)*, preferably first thing every morning and in a place with clean air. These positive actions along with the application of essential oils during massage can help to improve and prevent many complaints of the respiratory system.

The very breath we draw is dependent on how we care for our organs of respiration. Often, it is only when respiratory functions are impaired that we learn to appreciate them.

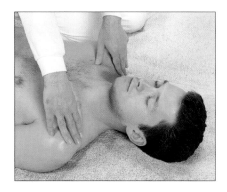

1 *Kneeling, feel for the space between the ribs in the upper chest. Starting from the breastbone, press with your thumbs, moving towards the shoulder. Repeat in the space beneath and continue until just above the breast area.*

2 *Covering the same area as in step 1, glide between the ribs using the heels of your hands. Keep the arms relaxed and let the motion come from your shoulders.*

3 *Using your thumbs rub the acupressure point LU 1 (see page 83), in an outward circular movement, for a minute or two. At first it might feel quite sore, but it will improve gradually.*

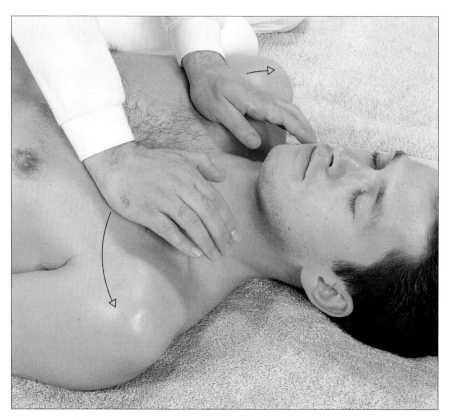

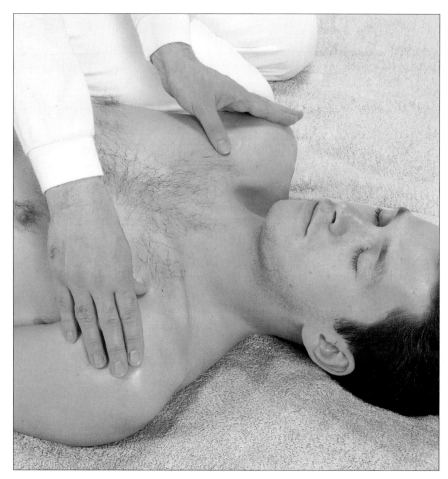

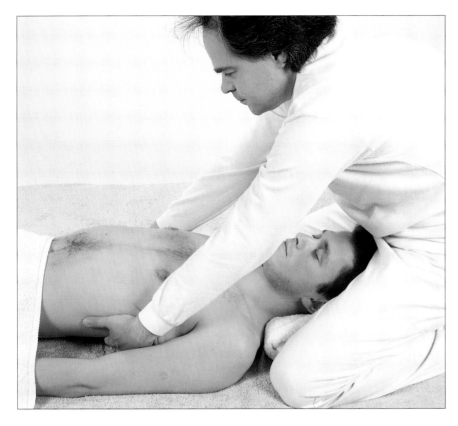

4 For the following three steps remember to always support your massage partner's head with a folded towel or a pillow. Kneel just above their head, bend slightly forward and place your two hands beneath the middle part of the recipient's back. Then gently but firmly pull the back up and towards you, creating a stretch of the chest and rib area. Hold this position for a few seconds, let go slowly and repeat the entire sequence two more times.

5 With the receiver lying on their left side, support the right arm just above the armpit, with your left hand, and slightly stretch it towards you. With your right hand push the rib cage in the opposite direction towards the feet. Hold for a few seconds; repeat twice. For upper, middle and lower portions of the rib cage.

6 Repeat the initial stages of step 5. Once you have stretched the rib cage with the left hand, use the thumb of the right hand to rub the intercostal muscles in the space between the ribs. This frees spasms in the rib muscles.

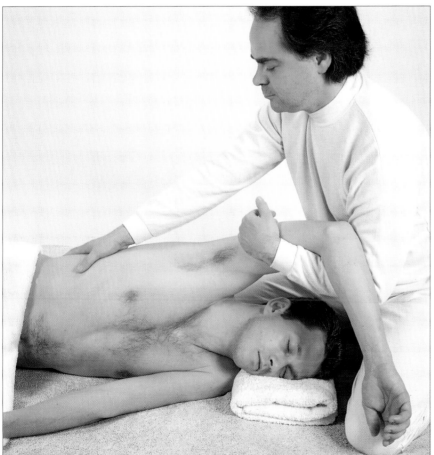

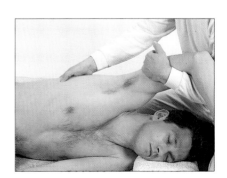

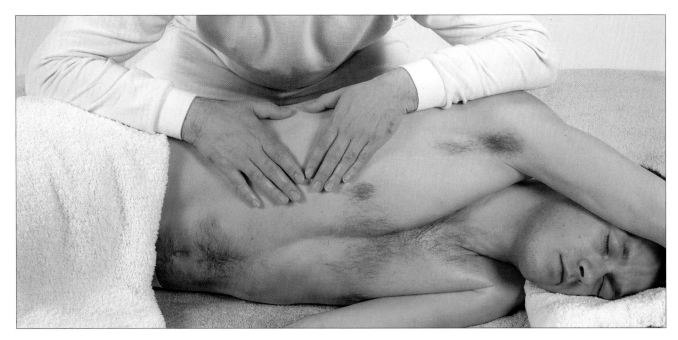

7 *Ask your partner to lie on their left side with their right arm stretched above their head, thus opening the right side of the rib cage. Kneel behind them and clasp their rib cage with the palms of both hands (see above). Your left hand pulls towards the receiver's head and the right towards their feet. This movement should be performed in the upper, middle and lower parts of the rib cage.*

Once you have performed steps 5, 6 and 7, repeat them on the other side of the body.

8 *Having massaged the ribs on the front of the body and the sides. Now turn the receiver on to their front and with your fingertips or thumbs rub between the rib spaces of the upper torso.*

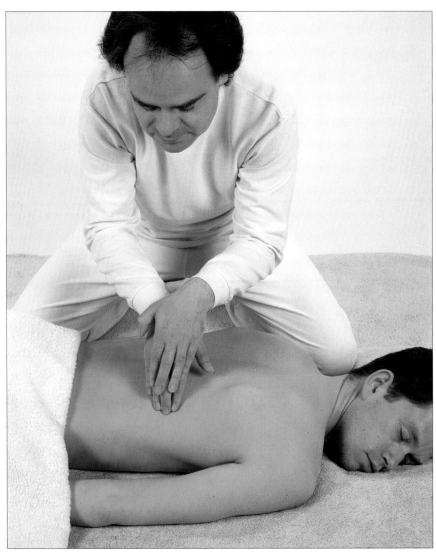

Self-help for Better Breathing

By treating yourself you will acquire a greater understanding of the techniques of massage, which will enhance your skill. The following breathing techniques have been selected because they are most suitable for self-massage and with practice can be learned by anyone, including the recipient for his or her own use. They will enable you to carry out a programme of self-help to bring both increased self-awareness and a feeling of well-being.

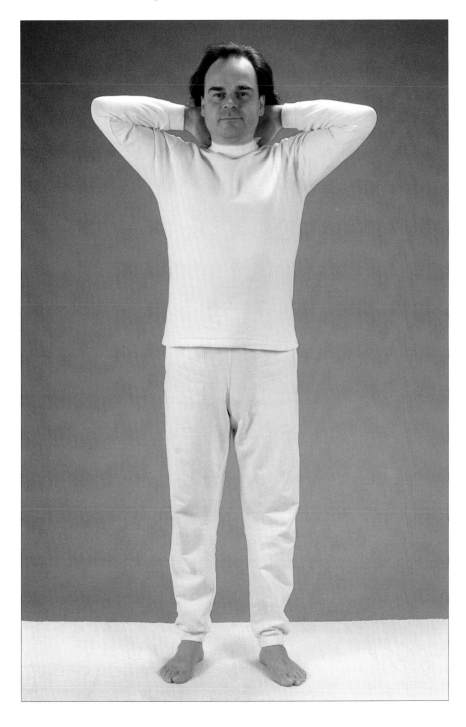

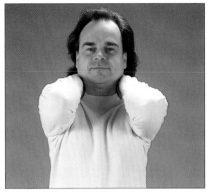

1 *Stand or sit with your hands clasped behind your neck and elbows facing forward* (see above). *Slowly breathe in stretching the elbows outwards to open the chest and allow a major intake of oxygen* (see left). *Then breathe out bringing the elbows forward to the starting position. Repeat four times.*

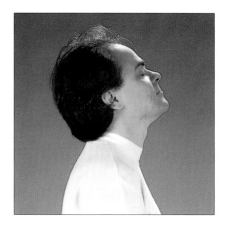

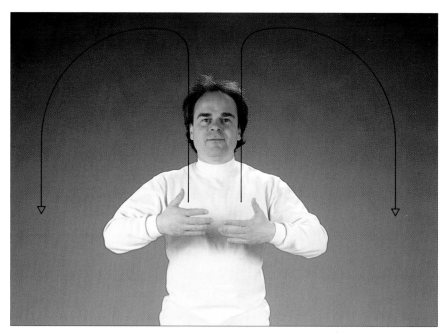

2 *This movement comes from the neck. Breathe in and slowly extend the neck backwards. Breathe out and slowly bring the neck forward towards your chest. Repeat. Repeat sequence four times.*

3 *Stand, and place your hands a short way away from your chest, the palms facing the body (see top right). Next start to slowly breathe in, raising your hands up and above your head with the palms facing the ceiling. Next start to breathe out, lowering your arms in a circular motion (see right) and bringing your hands back to the starting position. Repeat four times. Do not tense your neck or shoulders while performing it, and allow your breathing to flow slowly and evenly.*

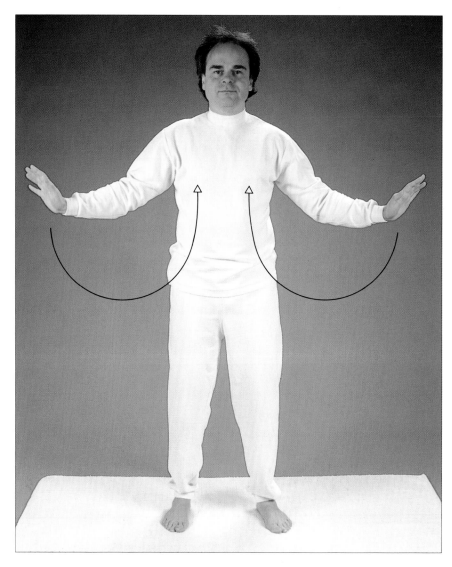

CHAPTER FIVE

Good Digestion

The function of the digestive system is to break down the food we eat, so that it can be absorbed and distributed to nourish the body. The massages, acupressure, self-help techniques and herbal teas in this chapter help to maintain good digestion, avoid digestive problems and enhance well-being.

The Digestive System

The digestive system works as follows: the food we swallow, propelled by peristalsis (muscular contractions), travels from the oesophagus (gullet) to the stomach, through the duodenum and into the small intestine where almost all the nutrients are absorbed. Whatever remains undigested passes through the large intestine (colon) and is excreted via the anus.

Essential aids to this digestive process are the liver, gall bladder and pancreas, which produce enzymes – powerful chemicals, that help to breakdown food.

Following are the four main stages that food undergoes in the digestive system.

Ingestion. The moment when food is taken in the mouth to be chewed and ground down into smaller particles by the teeth and movement of the jaws, and mixed with saliva, so that it can be swallowed via the pharynx and passes into the oesophagus (gullet) – the muscular tube-like passage – that runs down the centre of the chest to the stomach.

Saliva, which is part mucus, stimulates the taste-buds, helps to break down food, lubricates and protects the mouth from sharp particles and aids swallowing. It carries enzymes which start the breakdown of carbohydrates in food into easily assimilated sugars.

Digestion. This is the stage when the food

THE DIGESTIVE ORGANS

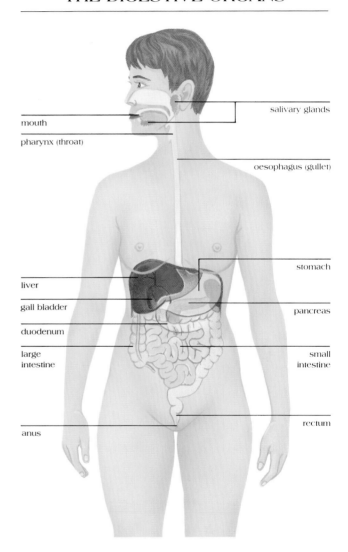

The digestive system, also known as the alimentary tract, consists of the mouth, pharynx (throat), oesophagus (gullet), stomach, small intestine (the duodenum, jejunum and ileum), and the large intestine (the caecum, colon and rectum). The associated digestive organs, which secrete digestive juices and break the food down as it passes through the digestive system, are the salivary glands, liver, gall bladder and pancreas.

remains in the stomach, while cells in the stomach walls begin the preliminary digestion process with hydrocholic acid, rennin, pepsin and lipase. The food then enters the small intestine, where it is further broken down by a complex chemical process performed by enzymes, digestive juices, pancreatic juices and bile from the liver.

Absorption. This is the process by which the digested substances, such as vitamins and minerals, pass through the walls of some of the areas of the alimentary canal to be distributed throughout the body.

Elimination. In this stage food substances that are no longer useful to the body are formed into a semi-solid waste matter in the large intestine, and are then excreted through the rectum and anus.

The time that food remains in the various stages of the digestive process, before being assimilated or excreted, is approximately as follows: about one minute in the mouth; ten-to-fifteen seconds in the oesophagus (gullet); up to four hours in the stomach; up to six hours in the small intestine; anything from ten hours to several days in the colon (large intestine).

Common Complaints

The pleasure of eating is too often marred by indigestion and other digestive problems. Fortunately, there are simple ways in which we can avoid or alleviate the discomforts commonly experienced after enjoying a meal.

Indigestion (dyspepsia)

This all-too-common complaint occurs when the digestive process is disrupted by the passage of food being obstructed, or the breakdown and absorption of nutrients being impeded.

Symptoms can include heartburn, aches and pains in the abdomen, nausea, and an excess of wind (flatulence) in the stomach or intestine. The latter results in belching and feeling bloated. If this happens often, we may also feel generally unwell. Persistent indigestion is often related to a stressful life style and an unbalanced diet.

If we eat when we are tense and in a hurry, our stomach is affected and food is not properly broken down, assimilated, and eliminated. The gastric juices then turn against the stomach creating inflammatory conditions and hyperacidity. Undigested food accumulates and stagnates in the intestines resulting in bloating and toxins with possible diarrhoea or constipation. The person often complains of feeling exhausted, irritable and confused and may also be unable to sleep.

ACUPRESSURE POINTS

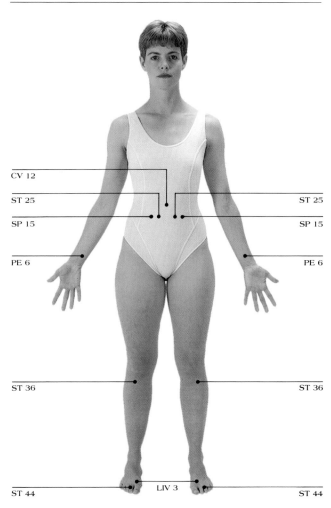

These acupressure points benefit the digestive system and help to strengthen digestive processes. They also soothe specific complaints: SP 15 eases constipation; ST 36 for indigestion; ST 44 for indigestion and constipation; ST 25 for irritable bowel syndrome and constipation; CV 12 to alleviate indigestion and nausea.

Prompt action, using the following self-help steps, can prevent chronic indigestion from leading to much more serious problems, such as colitis and ulcers. They can also help nausea, constipation and irritable bowel syndrome.

Eat at regular intervals, such as breakfast, lunch and dinner. And before eating, check your state of mind and body. If you are tense, make a conscious decision to relax by taking a few deep breaths.

Avoid an excess of stodgy or oily foods, such

ACUPRESSURE POINTS

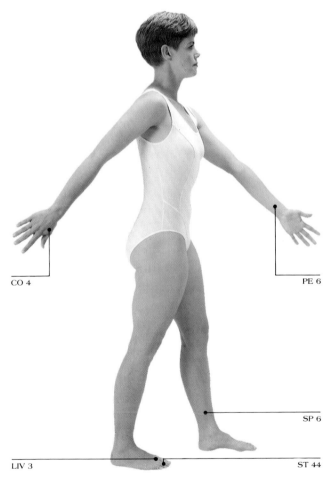

CO 4

PE 6

SP 6

LIV 3

ST 44

Other points encourage digestive functions. Each is also useful for certain complaints: CO 4 for indigestion, irritable bowel syndrome and constipation (do not use during pregnancy or with SP 6 if excessive menstrual flow); LIV 3 for indigestion, irritable bowel syndrome and billiousness; SP 6 for irritable bowel syndrome; PE 6 for irritable bowel syndrome and nausea.

as white bread, deep fried dishes, and full fat cheese. Choose, instead, whole grains, such as brown bread and brown rice, vegetables, pulses, white meat, fish and fresh fruit. Use the minimum of salt to avoid drinking too much while eating.

Do not overburden your stomach. Leave the table feeling satisfied, but still light.

The following acupressure points help digestion: ST 36, ST 44, CV 12 *(see page 92)*; CO 4 and LIV 3 *(see Chapter Three, page 72)*. Gently massage with a sedating motion each of these for two minutes three times a week.

Constipation

This term covers the discomfort caused by the infrequent and/or difficult passing of hard dry faeces (stools). Some people have sluggish bowels from birth, but for the majority of us constipation results from a sedentary life; faulty habits, such as not going to the lavatory when the body tells us to; and an inadequate diet. It can also be a symptom of an underlying disorder, requiring medical attention.

To alleviate constipation, avoid refined foods, such as white bread and sugar, and increase fibre, found in food, such as wholemeal bread and rice, and fresh fruit and vegetables. Try to take regular exercise. Add self-help bodywork techniques to your usual exercise.

Massage, using gentle rubbing strokes over the lower abdomen, performed either by a therapist or as self-massage *(see pages 97–8)*, will help peristalsis and the emptying of bowels. Massaging the following acupressure points with a circular motion, CO 4 *(see Chapter Three, page 72)*, SP 15, ST 25, ST 44, *(see page 92)* for two minutes each, three times a week, will also help.

Irritable bowel syndrome

Also known as spastic colon, this is a very common disorder of the lower bowel with intestinal tension, soreness and colicky pains. There could be constipation alternating with diarrhoea; distension (feeling bloated); flatulence (excessive wind); and agitation.

Although not life-threatening and unlikely

to lead to complications, the discomfort can be severe and distressing, often causing people to worry that they might have an attack of appendicitis or something of a more serious nature.

Irritable bowel syndrome can be avoided or brought under control through diet *(see page 91)*. During an acute episode, avoid stimulating drinks such as coffee and alcohol, foods that are hot and spicy, or fried; cakes; ice-creams; and acid-tasting fruits. Also avoid leaving the table feeling heavy and bloated.

Relaxation techniques, including the use of the breathing exercises *(see pages 87–8)*, and soothing massage are helpful.

Massaging the following acupressure points: SP 6, PE 6 *(see Chapter Two, page 55)*, LIV 3 *(see Chapter Three, page 72)*, ST 25 *(see below)* with a circular motion for two minutes three times a week, is also helpful.

HERBALS TEAS

Herbal teas are a pleasing way to soothe some digestive complaints. In each case infuse 5 mg (1 teaspoon) of the mixture in a cup of hot water for ten minutes. Strain and drink while warm. You can purchase mixtures for the following three teas in tincture form; add ten drops to half a glass of luke-warm water.

Indigestion. Drink the following tea, preferably after food. Mix, in equal parts, fennel seeds (*Foeniculum vulgare*), peppermint (*Metha piperita*), orange peel (*Citrus sinensis*) and marsh mallow root (*Althea officianalis*).

Constipation. After dinner or lunch and before retiring at night, drink a cup of the following tea. Mix together, in equal measures, liquorice (*Glycyrrhiza glabra*), marsh mallow root, fennel seeds and orange peel.

Irritable bowel syndrome. Drink one-to-two cups a day of the following tea. Mix, in equal parts, peppermint, aniseed (*Pimpinella anisum*), chamomile (*Chamaemelum nobile* syn. *Anthemis nobile*), liquorice and orange peel.

WARNING. For those who suffer from high blood pressure or fluid retention, use dandelion root (*Taraxacum officinale*) instead of liquorice for the above two teas.

Nausea. Mix, in equal parts, chamomile and aniseed.

Abdominal distension (bloating)
This is a generalized swelling of the abdomen that is not due to being overweight. Some causes need medical investigation, but most are harmless. However, wind in the body, stomach or intestine can be very uncomfortable.

Some women experience fluid retention, resulting in bloating of the lower abdomen, just before a menstrual period is due. If it is caused by digestive problems, the advice given under indigestion could alleviate the discomfort caused by abdominal distension. Constipation could also be a likely cause *(see page 91)*.

Nausea
A very uncomfortable feeling that you are going to vomit without necessarily doing so. This sensation may be accompanied by increased salivation, pallor and a cold sweat.

When the causes are due to a digestive problem or stress, massaging the acupressure points PE 6 *(see Chapter Two, page 55)* and CV 12 *(see below)* in a sedating manner.

ACUPRESSURE POINTS

The location of the points in this chapter are:

Spleen 15 (SP 15). Found four cuns on each side from the centre of the navel. SP 15 eases constipation.

Stomach 25 (ST 25). Located two cuns laterally from the centre of the navel. Eases irritable bowel syndrome, eases constipation.

Stomach 36 (ST 36). Found three cuns down from the crease of the knee to the shin bone (tibia) on the outside of the leg. It strengthens the whole body, helps digestion, relieves diarrhoea and pain in the knee.

Stomach 44 (ST 44). Found in the skin margin formed by the web between the second and third toes. Helps digestion, eases constipation.

Conception Vessel 12 (CV 12). Draw an imaginary line between the tip of the sternum (breastbone) and the navel; found half-way along. Strengthens digestion, calms nausea.

For PE 6 and SP 6 *(see Chapter Two, page 55)*; CO 4 and LIV 3 *(see Chapter Three, page 72)*.

Massage for Good Digestion

The gentle, relaxing, calming strokes used in the following massages soothe nerves, and are excellent ways to maintain good digestion and treat digestive problems. They also ease stomach aches commonly caused by stress and tension, and help to alleviate constipation. Before beginning the massage, study carefully the Digestive Organs diagram *(see page 89)*, so that you are familiar with the position of all the organs of the digestive system.

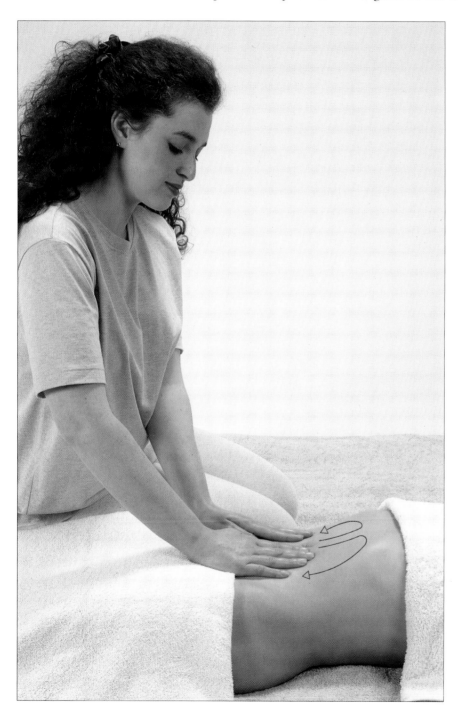

1 *Kneel alongside the receiver's hips* (see left), *place both hands together over the lower abdomen and, using a light pressure, massage upwards with both hands. When the tips of your fingers reach the breastbone, use your thumbs* (see below) *to massage under the entire rib cage area with a light-to-medium pressure. Glide your hands back to the navel, and continue lightly massaging the abdomen to the sides of the torso, returning in one smooth movement to the starting position. Repeat this slow soothing massage five times.*

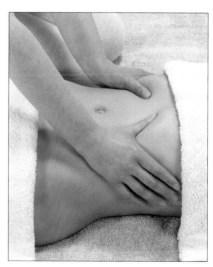

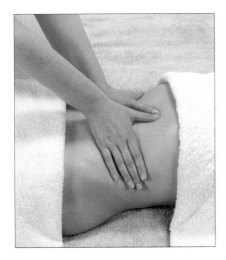

2 *The conception vessel meridian, runs along the centre of the abdomen. Start beneath the sternum using your thumbs apply pressure all the way down it. Repeat twice.*

3 *The area of the liver is just beneath the right rib cage. Using the heel of your hand, rub gently and rhythmically up and down with a light pressure, making sure that you cover the whole liver area (see right). Repeat a few times.*

4 *Using the heel of your hand, gently rub up and down the stomach area positioned just beneath the left rib cage. Repeat this sequence a few times.*
  This area – and the whole of the diaphragm area – which is positioned under the rib cage, is very prone to collecting tensions. Gentle rubbing and slow rhythmic stroking help to disperse tension, and soothe digestive problems.

MASSAGE OIL FOR INDIGESTION

Add to a saucer of 30 ml (2 tablespoons) of base oil, two drops of one essential oil – or one drop each of two essential oils – of orange, mandarin or grapefruit peels; peppermint, chamomile or aniseed.

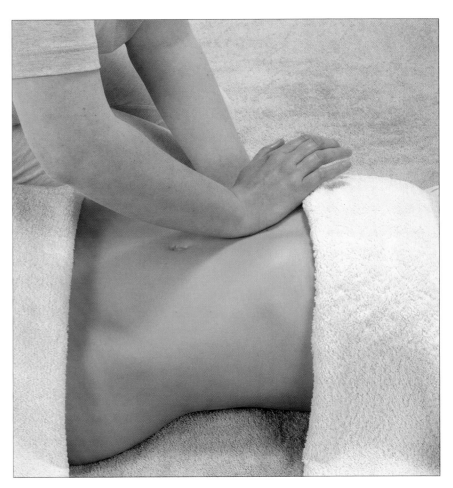

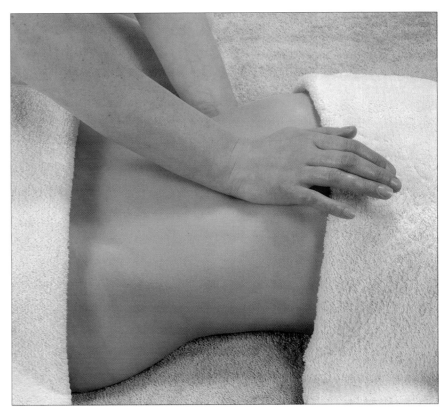

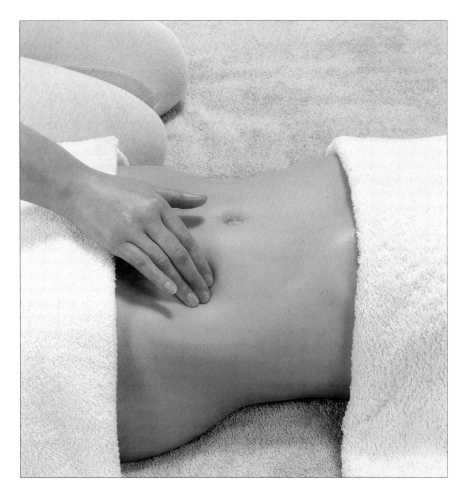

5 *Place the tips of your fingers in the area between the small and large intestine in the lower abdomen (see left). Breathe in deeply, and as you breathe out, gently rub, using a light but firm pressure, up to the navel and back in one movement. Repeat, slowly lowering your fingertips until you have massaged the whole of the small intestine area. Repeat this entire massage sequence for three minutes.*

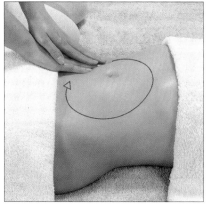

6 *Place one hand on top of the other (see above), keeping both relaxed, with your fingers flat against the lower part of the large intestine on the right side of the body. Using gentle pressure and circular, gliding strokes, work rhythmically across the transverse intestine all the way down to the lower part of the left side of the large intestine. Do this five times.*

7 *Using the heel of your hand, feel for contracted, hard tense areas along the large intestine tract. Continuing to use the heel of your hand, gently rub over these tense areas with a circular motion until you feel the area relax. Do not rub for more than two minutes in one spot, and do not treat more than three spots in one session. Do not press hard, and stop at once if there is any discomfort.*

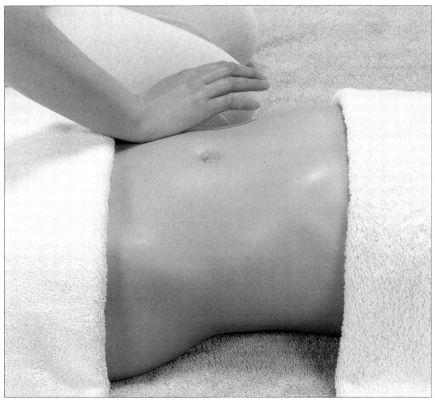

MASSAGE OIL FOR CONSTIPATION

Massage the abdomen, particularly the large intestinal area with the following massage oil: 30 ml (2 tablespoons) of base oil to which you have added one drop of essential oils of fennel and orange peel.

8 *Kneel down opposite your partner's abdomen (see right). Then, place both your palms flat over the abdomen. Breathe in and, as you breathe out, start the massage, using alternate hands to gently rub the flesh from side to side on the abdomen. The emphasis here is more on pulling up over the side of the abdomen than pressing down. Continue for one minute.*

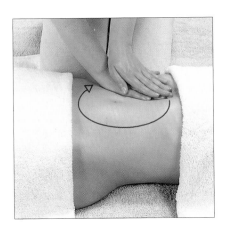

9 *Put one hand on top of the other on the lower right of the abdomen (see above). Breathe in and, as you breathe out, start effleuraging the whole of the abdomen area using a moderate pressure in a circular and rhythmical motion. Perform seven circles in a continuous movement.*

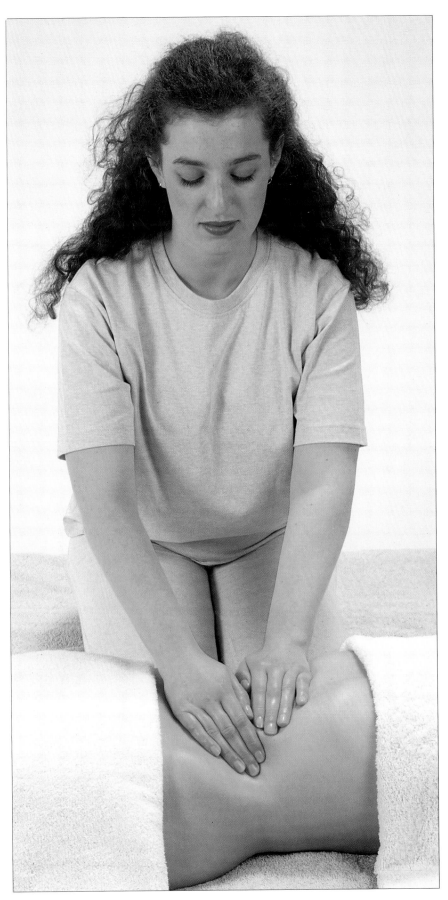

Self-help for Good Digestion

If practised regularly for a few minutes three times a week, these massage exercises can release abdominal tension, often the cause of minor but debilitating digestive complaints.

If your digestion is good, practise the following massages only once a week. If you suffer from an acute or chronic digestive complaint, consult your practitioner about the suitability of these self-help techniques. Leave at least two hours between a meal and the massage.

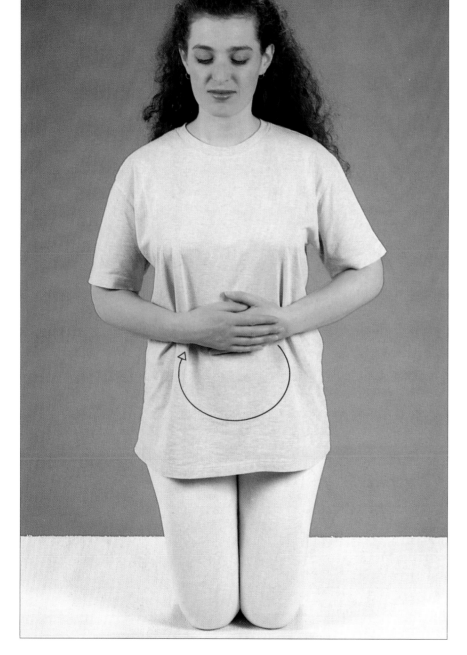

1 *Kneeling or standing, place one hand on top of the other on the lower right of the abdomen. Breathe in and, as you breathe out, start rubbing the whole abdomen in a circular rhythmical motion (see left), using a moderate pressure. Perform fifteen circles.*

2 *Carry out the same technique as above, but this time concentrate the moderate-pressure rub on the large intestine area (see below), which surrounds the lower abdomen. Perform twenty-five circles in a continually flowing, rhythmical movement.*

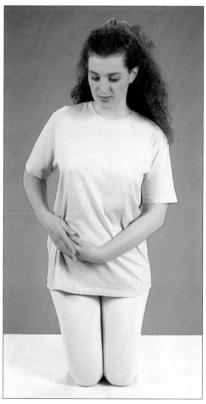

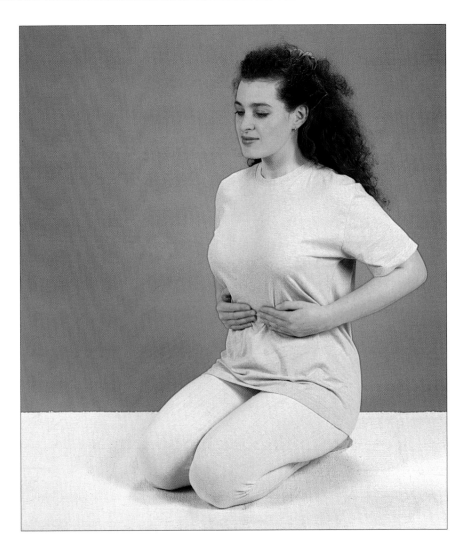

3 *Sit on your heels and place the palm of your hands over your upper abdomen above the navel (see above right). Take a deep breath and, while breathing out, bend forward (see below right) without lifting your torso. Remain bent for about ten seconds breathing regularly. In this position your palms will gently compress your abdomen. Repeat the whole sequence once more, but this time place your palms on your lower abdomen.*

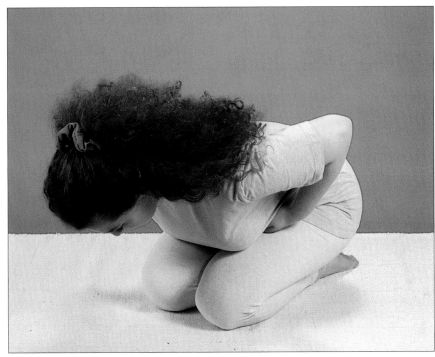

CHAPTER SIX

Clean Water

The urinary system performs the vital functions of cleansing our blood of waste products and expelling them from the body in the urine. It comprises the kidneys, where urine is produced, the ureter tubes, which carry the urine away from the kidneys, the bladder where the urine is stored, and the urethra, which empties the bladder outside the body. These vital organs lie just above the waist at the back of the abdominal cavity, below the liver on the right and the spleen on the left.

The Urinary System

The kidneys filter our blood, absorbing fluids, nutrients and toxins, to maintain a constant balance in our system and make urine from these waste products. Through the urine the kidneys eliminate excessive fluid concentration and waste material. From the kidneys it is transported to the bladder via the ureter tubes for storage. When the bladder is full the urethra carries the urine to the exterior. During stress and nervousness blood pressure rises, stimulating the kidneys to eliminate quantities of water, increasing the volume of urine.

To fully appreciate the action of the kidneys, remember that the body is composed primarily of water, ranging from 45 to 75 per cent of body weight, depending on the amount of fat present and age. Maintaining the correct fluid balance is necessary for our survival.

Common Complaints

Many illnesses involve the urinary system, particularly the kidneys. Most complaints, because of their critical and complex nature, are beyond the scope of this book. However, the self-help

THE URINARY ORGANS

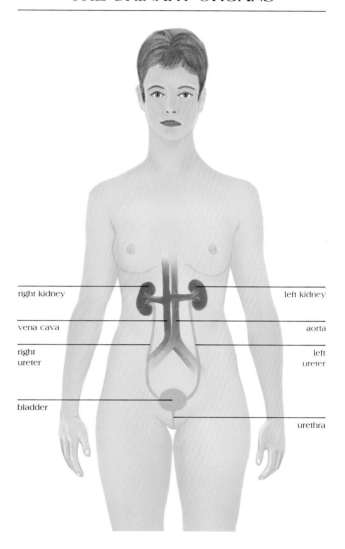

right kidney

left kidney

vena cava

aorta

right
ureter

left
ureter

bladder

urethra

Urine is formed and excreted via the urinary system. Each kidney has about one million filtering units where blood is filtered to make urine. The urine collects in the renal pelvises (ducts that channel urine from the kidneys) and is then carried by peristalsis, the wave-like contractions in the muscular ureter walls, down the ureter tubes to the bladder where it is stored until expelled through the urethra.

massage techniques and advice here can help strengthen the kidneys and prevent weakness.

Cystitis and Urethritis

These two very common and similar conditions can be treated along the same lines. Cystitis relates to inflammation of the inner lining of the bladder, urethritis to inflammation of the urethra. Symptoms can be mild or severe, transient or lasting over a long period of time. There could be one episode, but often it tends to recur. In both conditions the urine tends to be too acidic. This causes pain and burning or stinging when passing urine, due to inflammation in the urethra and bladder. There is an urgent and frequent need to pass urine, often when there is very little. It might contain a cloudy sediment, even blood. Other symptoms may include both discomfort and pain in the lower abdomen.

A combination of causes, particularly for urethritis, could be: cold weather, various irritants, clothing that is too tight or tampons. However, it is thought that the main cause is bacteria, either contracted during intercourse or originating from the anal passage after evacuation of stools. These complaints affect women more than men, because of the proximity of the female urethra opening (in front of the vagina) to the anus and because the female urethra is much shorter, making it easier for bacteria to get to the bladder.

One preventive step advised by doctors, particularly in Anglo-Saxon countries, is to always wipe the anus away from rather than towards the genitals. My advice is to wipe backwards first and then wash the anal area with water and neutral soap after each evacuation.

During attacks of cystitis avoid all foods that tend to inflame and create acidity, such as spicy food, white bread, fried food, red meat, dairy products, coffee and alcohol. Eat more whole grains, fresh vegetables, fish, some fruits in moderation but avoiding citruses.

Although massage can help in alleviating some of the most distressing symptoms, do not practise it directly on the bladder during an

ACUPRESSURE POINTS

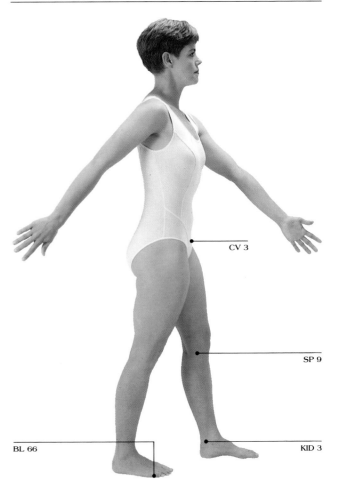

The acupressure points shown in this diagram are all useful for urinary problems. More specifically, CV 3 can alleviate cystitis and urethritis; SP 9 is useful for urinary infections; KID 3 strengthens low vitality and BL 66 is helpful for cystitis. Massage these points with circular pressure as part of a body massage or treat several times a week as required.

BARLEY WATER FOR CYSTITIS AND URETHRITIS

Barley water is very useful for soothing inflammation and relieving pain. Some commercial preparations contain too much sugar and too many chemicals. Prepare your own by simmering 50 g (2 oz) of barley in 1 litre (1¾ pint) of water for 40 minutes. Strain and add a few drops of lemon. Drink this barley water over a period of 24 hours.

EASING CYSTITIS WITH ESSENTIAL OILS

The following combination of essential oils can bring relief to cystitis even during an acute attack: to a saucer of 30 ml (2 tablespoons) of base oil add two drops of lavender, one of sandalwood and one of tea-tree; massage some on the bladder area once or twice a day. You can also massage in the lower back particularly around the sacrum. Do not massage over the urinary bladder during an episode of acute discomfort.

acute attack. Instead massage the lower back and other areas. Massaging the lower back can soothe the nerves that control the genital area. *(See also Chapter One, page 34–43 for specific massage techniques that would be useful.)*

If you suspect you have cystitis or urethritis, always consult a doctor.

Low vitality

If you feel lethargic with little motivation and your lower back feels weak, cold, sore and lacking in strength, you might be suffering from what Chinese medicine calls 'weak kidney Yang'. Other symptoms are copious, pale urine and lack of sexual drive. Warm and tone the lower back area with essential oils such as juniper, rosemary or ginger.

If you have the above symptoms, but get hot and sweaty during the night and your urine is scant and red, you might be suffering from 'weak kidney Yin'. Cool and tone the lower back with essential oils of rose, geranium or vetiver.

Acupressure Points

The following points are beneficial in easing some urinary system problems. Massage by rubbing in a circular motion with your thumb, using a gentle but constant pressure and always communicating a sense of warmth.

Conception vessel 3 (CV 3). Find the middle of the pubic bone: a little bony promontory just where the lower abdomen curves towards the genitals. Draw an imaginary line between this point and the navel. CV 3 is on this line one cun above the pubic bone. This point lies above the bladder and it is used to help most conditions associated with this organ like cystitis, and genito-urinary problems like urethritis.

Spleen 9 (SP 9). On the inner side of both legs, follow the tibia (the large bone in the front of the lower leg); when it reaches the knee it curves. Massage the fleshy part next to the middle of this curve. Used for urinary infections.

KID 3 strengthens low vitality. *(See Chapter Three, page 72.)*

BL 66 is used for painful conditions of the bladder. *(See Chapter One, page 33.)*

Massage for Clean Water

As we have learned, massage with the appropriate essential oils can help allay some physical complaints of the urinary system such as cystitis and urethritis and the mental distress often accompanying them. Ever popular lavender is calming and improves circulation; it can be used every day for acute conditions, but do not use it for more than two consecutive weeks because of its sedative qualities. Sandalwood is widely used for urinary infections because of its anti-inflammatory and soothing nature and it also promotes peace of mind, which aids recovery. Tea-tree is noted for its action against bacteria, fungi and viruses, making it effective in allaying cystitis.

For 'weak kidney Yang' *(see above)* juniper is a stimulating essential oil, but not recommended for acute inflammation of the kidneys; rosemary stimulates and warms; ginger is useful for warming the body and alleviating fatigue.

For 'weak kidney Yin' *(see above)* rose essential oil is beneficial; geranium is soothing and balancing; vetiver is good for circulation and gives a pleasant sense of languor.

1 *With the tips of the fingers gently massage in a circular motion over the bladder area for about one minute. In people who suffer from urinary infections you might feel some grainy sediments – like rubbing your fingers over sand. As the condition improves these disappear.*

2 *With the heel of the hand, massaging gently and slowly, rub up and down the bladder area for about one minute. The pressure should be gentle but constant.*

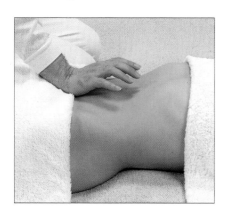

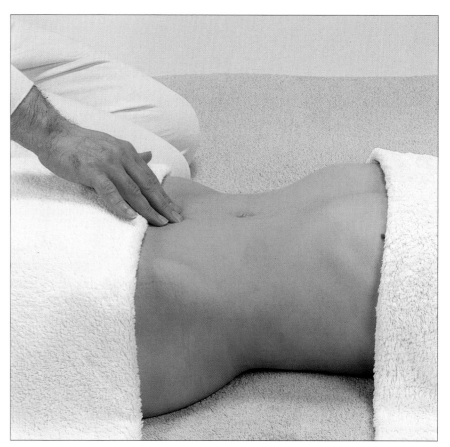

3 *Locate the reflex point of the kidneys in the sole of the foot (see below). Using the thumb rub in a circular motion. Then glide along the ureter tube reflex (see right); rub the bladder reflex. Repeat three times a week until symptoms ease, then once a week.*

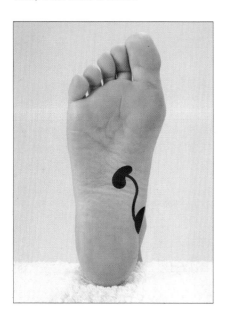

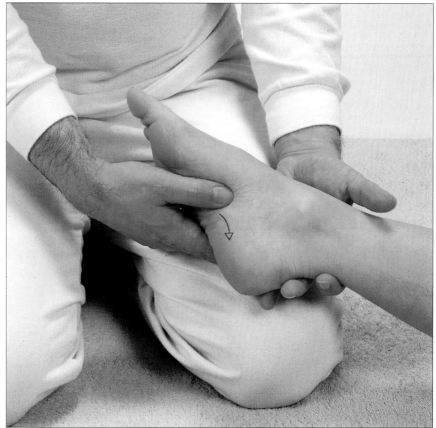

Self-help for Clean Water

Remember that the techniques described in this section to help the kidney area, also complement the self-help section under the back; they all help to keep the lower back healthy and supple. The kidney exercises following help to endow the back with strength.

By regularly stimulating the kidneys and massaging the bladder area, we can contribute to preventing many recurring and distressing urinary problems. These techniques also encourage proper elimination of the body's waste products in the urine through the urinary system.

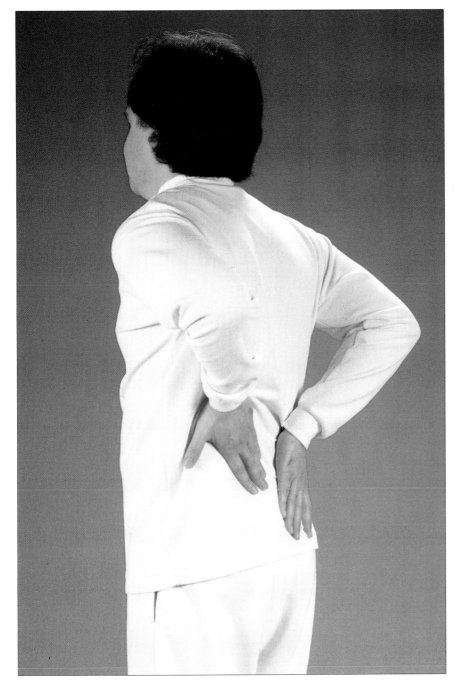

1 In a standing position, rub the kidney and lower back area with the open palms of your hands for a few minutes or until you experience a pleasant sensation of warmth.

2 With very loose fists gently percuss over the kidney and lower back area for a minute or two – a good way to revitalize ourselves. Do not percuss too strongly.

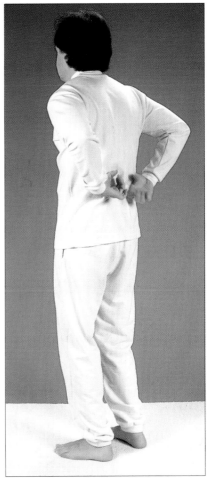

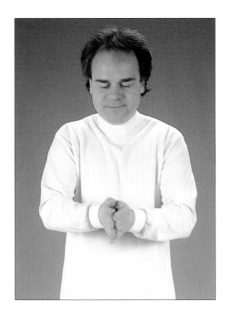

3 *Rub the palms of your hands together until they feel quite warm* (see above). *Then place one hand on top of the other over the bladder* (see right) *and as the warmth radiates to it, it will begin to feel warm and healthy. When the hands feel cold again you can repeat the exercise twice more.*

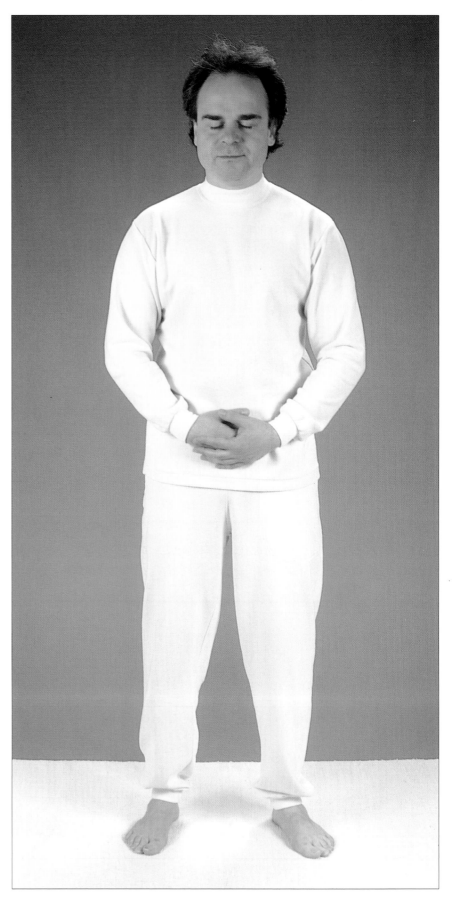

CHAPTER SEVEN

Reproductive Issues

Sexual activity is basic to all living creatures. A focal point of pleasure and strong emotions with all their contradictions, this activity ensures that reproduction occurs and the species survives in a new generation. During puberty the reproductive organs and glands begin to develop; this is the beginning of adulthood. The sensitive female reproductive organs are much more complex than the male. Massage, with its caring touch, and bodywork, aimed at building a healthier, stronger body, can enhance immeasurably this side of the lives of both sexes. The beauty of massage is that it can bring great closeness, no matter what our age.

Female Issues

A finely tuned timing mechanism controls the major physical female processes of menstruation, conception, pregnancy and the menopause. Massage can help to keep the female reproductive system healthy and give comfort when there are problems.

The Female Reproductive System

The internal female reproductive organs are the vagina, the uterus (womb), two fallopian tubes (the uterine tubes), and two ovaries. The vagina is a tubular organ which acts as a passage that connects the external genitalia and the internal reproductive organs. It releases uterine fluids and the menstrual flow; it receives the seminal fluid from the male; and it serves as the lower end of the birth canal.

The uterus is a hollow muscular organ shaped like a pear, lying between the urinary bladder and the rectum. Following the onset of puberty, the uterus goes through a regular monthly cycle, the menstrual cycle, in order to receive, nourish and protect a fertilized ovum. At about the middle of each menstrual cycle the ovaries produce an ovum that can be fertilized when it enters into contact with a male sperm.

If fertilized it then deposits itself in the lining of the uterus and pregnancy begins. The uterus is the environment for the growing fetus.

The ovaries are two glands resembling two large almonds each weighing about 3 g (⅛ oz). They are located on either side of the uterus, and produce the all important female sex hormones oestrogen and progesterone. These hormones are needed to bring about normal sexual development and the healthy functioning of the female reproductive system. The ovaries in turn are controlled by hormones produced by the pituitary gland in the brain.

The uterine tubes convey the ovum from the ovaries to the uterus, so we sometimes hear that a woman has difficulty in conceiving because of blocked fallopian tubes.

The Menstrual Cycle

The monthly cycle regulates the lining of the uterus (the endometrium), which increases in thickness in order to receive and nourish a fertilized egg. The cycle is controlled by various hormones secreted by the ovaries and the pituitary gland. If conception does not take place, the production of hormones from the ovaries

FEMALE REPRODUCTIVE SYSTEM

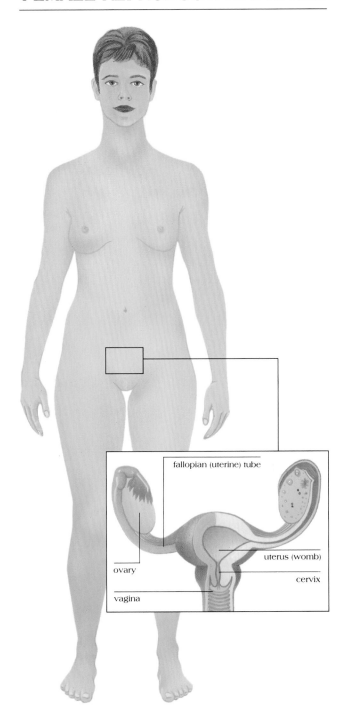

The female reproductive system consists of the organs that enable a woman to ovulate, to have sexual intercourse, to nourish a fertilized ovum and to give birth. Shown here, partly in cross-section, are the internal genitalia: two ovaries which produce and release one ovum or egg per cycle; two uterine tubes, where fertilization occurs; the uterus where the fetus grows; the cervix; and the vagina.

diminishes for the time being. The lining of the uterus which is not needed is then shed. Uterine contractions force the menstrual blood to be expelled into the vagina. Blood loss varies from person to person, even from cycle to cycle; the average is 60 ml (2 fl oz).

Common Complaints

Massage is particularly beneficial in improving several complaints related to the female reproductive system, for the menstrual cycle often brings discomfort and marked mood swings due to changes in hormonal activity.

Premenstrual Tension (PMT) and Painful Periods (dysmenorrhoea)

These two conditions seem to affect a large proportion of women. They are mainly attributed to irregularities within the delicate framework of hormones that govern the female reproductive cycle. The physical and emotional symptoms of PMT may include a bloated feeling, irritability, depression and tension.

Painful and irregular periods are often indicated by a cramp-like pain or discomfort in the lower abdomen with nausea or vomiting.

The following advice applies to PMT and painful periods as the two are often related.

Massage and bodywork when administered as self-help, coupled with other natural ways, can be of help in alleviating problems.

Besides the massage techniques described in this section, massage can be useful in relaxing

RELIEF FOR PMT WITH HERBAL TEA

This tea can also bring some relief. Mix in equal parts the following herbs: marigold flowers *(Calendula officinalis)*, chamomile *(Chamaemelum nobile* syn. *Anthemis nobile)*, lemon balm *(Melissa officinalis)* and cramp bark *(Viburnum opulus)*. Make a tea by infusing 5 ml (1 teaspoon) of the mixture for ten minutes in a cup of hot water. Strain before drinking and have one or two cups a day at least one week before a period and continue till the second day of the period or if required till the end of menstruation.

> ## MASSAGE OIL FOR PMT
> To a saucer of 30 ml (2 tablespoons) of base oil, add one drop each of the following essential oils: lavender, chamomile and orange peel or geranium.

ACUPRESSURE POINTS

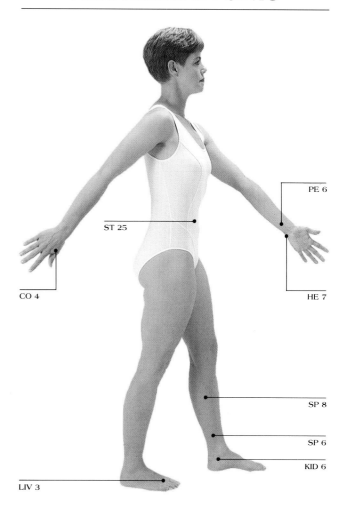

The acupressure points illustrated above are all useful for female reproductive problems. SP 8, PE 6 and ST 25 all alleviate painful periods; CO 4 and LIV 3 are useful for PMT; HE 7, SP 6 and KID 6 are helpful in alleviating symptoms of the menopause, KID 6 is good for night sweats. See relevant chapters for exact location.

the person and in regulating many body processes. If the woman is in pain and discomfort massaging areas like the hands and feet (*see Chapter Two, page 51*) and the head (*see Chapter Eight, page 113*) can be beneficial. Rubbing the lower back could bring relief due to organ innervation originating from the spine.

Premenstrual tension can also be relieved with acupressure. At least one week before the period is due massage once a day for two minutes each the following points: CO 4 and LIV 3 (*see Chapter Three, page 72*), SP 8 (*see page 108*). Keep massaging these points until the second day of the period. For abdominal cramps during the period: PE 6 (*see Chapter Two, page 55*) and ST 25 (*see Chapter Five, page 92*).

Many women swear by the beneficial effects of diet and supplements. It is advisable, particularly close to the period, to avoid coffee and to cut down on alcohol and sugar. Evening primrose oil and vitamins B6 and B complex are also useful; ask your health food shop or therapist to advise you on dosages.

Excessive menstrual flow (menorrhagia)
This could be due to an imbalance of the oestrogen and progesterone hormones, or growths like polyps and fibroids, but in many cases the cause is unknown. It is best not to massage over the abdomen or in the lower back, especially during the period. Instead massage the head, shoulders and limbs.

Menopause
This phase of a woman's life occurs between the ages of 45 and 55 when the ovaries reduce their production of oestrogen hormones. This can cause physical and psychological changes. While some women go through the menopause virtually symptom-free, a large percentage do experience various degrees of discomfort which may require radical attention. The lack of oestrogen may cause: hot flushes and night sweats, vaginal dryness, poor memory, anxiety, changes in metabolism and osteoporosis, among others. The symptoms occur with varying frequency and severity. The menopause, of course, is not an illness although many texts seem to refer to it as such. It is a life change and like all processes of transformation needs to be assisted and facilitated.

ESSENTIAL OILS FOR THE MENOPAUSE

The massage treatment should aim to be soothing and relaxing thus promoting restful sleep, tranquillity and good circulation. Use the following essential oils. Add two or three drops of a single one, or one drop each of three different ones, to 30 ml (2 tablespoons) of base oil: lavender, geranium, vetiver, neroli, chamomile, cypress, orange peel, mandarin peel, clary sage. (*See also Insomnia in Chapter Nine, page 140*).

Treatment includes massage, bodywork and particularly acupressure. All can be beneficial for those conditions with symptoms like hot flushes with circulatory problems, night sweats, restlessness, insomnia and palpitations.

Chinese medicine views such menopausal changes as a reduction in the Yin energy of the body and a resulting excess of Yang energy. Because the Yin energy cools and relaxes the body while the Yang warms and activates, the person is likely to experience excessive heat and restlessness. The acupressure points recommended (*see below*) aim to alleviate the symptoms of this imbalance.

Symptoms of the menopause can also be eased with certain acupressure points. KID 6 should be massaged with a toning technique; press on the points for a few seconds and release; repeat five times. Other acupressure points can be treated with a more calming technique: SP 6 (*see Chapter Two, page 55*); LIV 3 (*see Chapter Three, page 72*); HE 7 (*see below*). All are invaluable in easing these complaints.

Female frigidity
See instructions for male impotence, page 110.

Acupressure Points

The following points are helpful in easing complaints of the female reproductive system.

Spleen 8 (SP 8). With the knee flexed, the point is three cuns down from the crease of the knee on the inner leg next to the tibia. This main point for painful periods and menstrual cramps favours a smooth circulation of blood in the uterus and lower abdomen.

Heart 7 (HE 7). Found on the very end of the wrist crease on the side of the little finger; calming and soothing point good for nervous complaints like insomnia, anxiety, restlessness.

Kidney 6 (KID 6). Find the tip of the inner ankle bone. This point is one cun directly below it. It strengthens the kidneys and adrenals. It is particularly useful when there is excessive dryness in the body due to a kidney weakness. It is a cooling and moistening point, useful for hot conditions such as night sweats and hot flushes.

The location descriptions for other useful acupressure points can be found as follows: CO 4, SP 6, ST 25, and ST 36 (*see Chapter Five, page 92*); PE 6 (*see Chapter Nine, page 140*). (*See also Acupressure under Male Reproductive Issues, see page 111*).

Massage for Female Issues

Essential oils and massage soothe tension and other forms of nervous discomfort. They also promote good circulation, allaying problems like hot flushes, hot or cold extremities and abdominal cramps. In China it is believed that acupressure points can to a certain extent harmonize hormonal irregularities. Their use can help to regulate the flow of energy and the balance between Yin and Yang.

Many women with reproductive difficulties who have used natural and soothing techniques, such as massage and aromatherapy, have reported an improvement.

Massage and bodywork in general can be of help in the discomfort caused by hormonal irregularities. The self-help techniques, and a good diet, can soothe the abdomen in general and therefore the inner reproductive area.

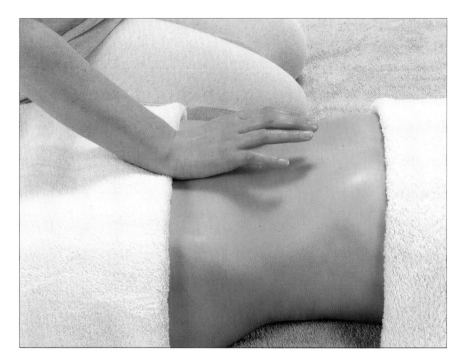

1 *Kneeling alongside the receiver's abdomen, place the heel of the hand just above the urinary bladder area. Using a light pressure, rub slowly over a space of only 5 cm (2 in) corresponding to the uterine area. Do not use this massage during menstruation.*

2 *With one hand on top of the other gently rub the lower abdominal area in a clockwise circular motion. Concentrate on relaxing and communicating warmth to the area. Do not use this during menstruation.*

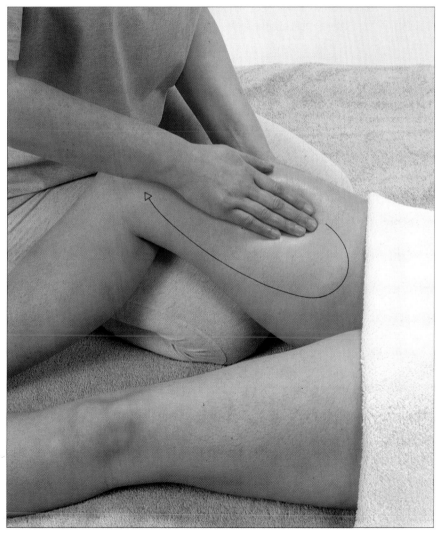

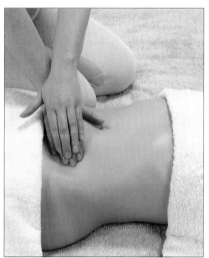

3 *Kneeling, facing the receiver, slightly flex their leg resting the knee and thigh over your thigh. Massage up and down the inner thigh with an open palm in a soothing fashion. The stroke should be smooth and continuous with a light to medium pressure. This technique can often bring relief to menstrual cramps.*

Male Issues

The male reproductive system is designed to produce sperm for the sake of reproduction. Problems are a matter of great concern to the individual. Massage, with the deep sense of relaxation it brings, allows body systems to regulate and regenerate themselves. The latter is difficult for the body to do if one is in a state of hyper-activity or anxiety.

The Male Reproductive System

The main components of the male reproductive system are the penis, the testes (testicles), the vas deferens (sperm ducts), the ejaculatory ducts, the prostate gland and the urethra. The testes, held in the scrotum, manufacture sperm and secrete the hormone testosterone which governs male characteristics such as tighter skeletal formation, more extensive hair growth pattern, greater muscular development and deeper voice.

The two vas deferens are sperm ducts that lead from the epididymis or spermatic cord (where sperm is stored and slowly matures) to the seminal vesicles and urethra. The vas deferens are cut during a vasectomy.

The main functions of the male reproductive system are to produce and convey sperm in order to fertilize the female ovum.

Common Complaints

Problems with genitalia, sometimes of a minor nature, are of great concern to most men. While the reasons may be physical, there may also be a psychological aspect. Here massage can help to relax and give confidence.

Impotence

Many experts consider that at some stage most men will experience a degree of impotence or lack of erectile vigour. Unless there is a clear health problem like diabetes, impotence is

MALE REPRODUCTIVE SYSTEM

The external male reproductive organs are the penis and the scrotum which holds the two testes. The main internal reproductive organs are as shown in the inset. Sperm produced from the testes passes along the vas deferens to the prostate gland and urethra. Fluid is added and the resulting semen ejaculated.

bladder

vas deferens

penis

urethra

testis

prostate gland

scrotum

often attributed to stress, fatigue or lack of self-confidence. Any male (or female) who is undergoing a period of over-work, emotional trauma or deep-seated feeling of anxiety or guilt could experience an episode of weak sexual drive. The fear of its repetition and anxiety can transform an isolated episode into a semi-permanent emotional and sexual blockage.

The approach below eases tension while increasing vitality. Practise this acupressure at least three times a week for three months. Acupressure for impotence or frigidity: with your thumb press continuously for a few seconds and then release the pressure to repeat again three times the following three points: KID 3 (*see Chapter Three, page 72*); ST 36 (*see Chapter Five, page 92*); and CV 6 (*see page 112*).

ESSENTIAL OILS FOR IMPOTENCE OR FRIGIDITY

In a saucer of 30 ml (2 tablespoons) of base oil, add one drop each of the essential oils of ylang-ylang, juniper and sandalwood. Otherwise just add three drops of the essential oil of jasmine, in my experience by far the best aphrodisiac oil.

If tension is present gently rub for a minute each PE 6 (*see Chapter Two, page 55*); and HE 7 (*see page 108*).

Premature Ejaculation

This occurs when the semen is ejected too soon on sexual arousal. Massage can benefit this condition, as it is often connected with organic and mental nervous hypersensitivity.

It is very important that the person experiencing this condition should learn how to relax thoroughly and breathe slowly and harmoniously (*see The Preparation, page 23*). Before sexual contact the man should have a few minutes of relaxation. During the act he should keep his musculature as relaxed as possible, his breathing even and deep. This will help to avoid over arousal and premature ejaculation.

Massage releases tension and anxiety and at the same time stimulates a low vitality. Refer also to the techniques for the lower back section (*pages 34 and 112*), to stimulate the lower abdomen and genital functions. If the person is very tense, refer also to Chapter Nine (*page 138*).

Massage mainly with soothing and calming strokes with relaxing essential oils such as lavender, chamomile, and neroli. Until alleviated, avoid the stimulating techniques.

While lying with his partner he should concentrate on the pleasurable feelings of intimacy and touch rather than on intercourse. When it happens it should arise from feelings of both joy and calmness.

Acupressure Points

Use of the following acupressure points can be of some benefit to a variety of worrying male

ACUPRESSURE POINTS

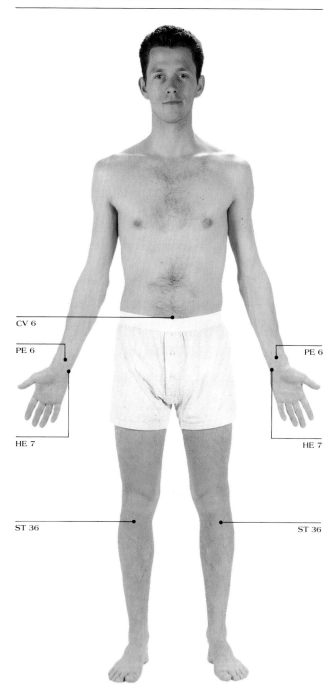

Massaging these acupressure points can calm and tone the body and strengthen sexual drive and endurance. All the acupressure points illustrated above are particularly useful in alleviating male impotence, for they help relax and give confidence. Massage ST 36, CV 6 and KID 3 (see page 72) by pressing with your thumb for a few seconds, releasing and repeating three times. Rub PE 6 and HE 7 gently with your thumb for a minute each. Do this three times a week for three months.

reproductive problems, especially impotence.

Conception Vessel 6 (CV 6). The point is located on the midline of the abdomen one and a half cuns beneath the navel. CV 6 is a very good point when dealing with weakness, lethargy and poor endurance because it will tone up and strengthen the recipient's body to give him both renewed vigour and confidence.

Several other acupressure points can be helpful in easing common and distressing problems of the male reproductive system. PE 6 (*see Chapter Two, page 55*); KID 3 (*see Chapter Three, page 72*); ST 36 (*see Chapter Five, page 92*); and HE 7 (*see page 108*).

Massage for Male Issues

In male problems there is often a combination of mental stress and tension which can lead to debility. The traditional approach, particularly in China, states that when tension is accompanied with debility, first relax, then tone. Massage relaxes the muscles of the upper back when they are unduly contracted, while promoting circulation and vigour in the genital area. This advice is valid for both men and women. Follow the massage sequence for the back (*see Chapter One, page 34*) and include the two steps below where appropriate.

1 *Using the heels of both hands alternately in a gentle rhythmic way, and using moderate vigour, rub up and down the sacral area. This action creates a gentle and pleasant sensation of warmth.*

2 *Using both hands, squeeze and lift the buttocks in a rhythmic fashion using alternate hands. Grab the flesh with the thumb flexed behind the four fingers, the squeeze should be firm enough to lift the area but not so tight as to hurt. The buttocks are often omitted during massage; however, they are formed by large muscles that can, due to their attachments to the pelvis, contribute to lower back problems affecting circulation in the genital area.*

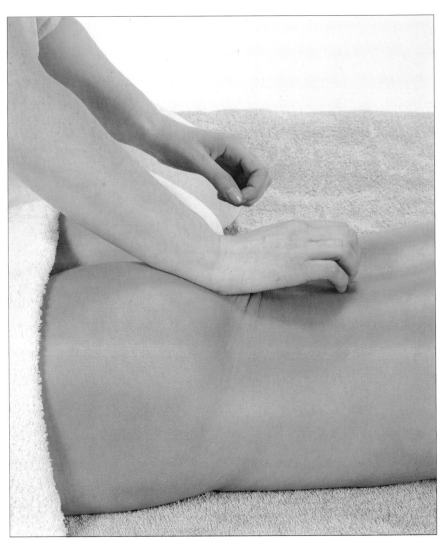

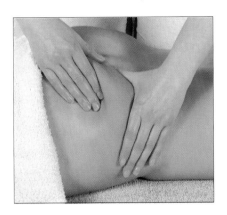

CHAPTER EIGHT

A Clear Head

In this chapter we deal with the uppermost part of the body which comprises the neck, skull and face. These very important areas can benefit greatly from massage. It can improve circulation in the head and face and relax the muscles of the neck. Massaging these places is not only a very pleasurable exercise but it is also immensely therapeutic, alleviating some conditions such as headaches, migraines, sinusitis, whiplash and torticollis (wry neck).

There are other notable benefits: massage increases lymphatic drainage from the head, expulsion of mucus from the sinuses, and circulation to the face and skull, which helps to give the recipient a youthful complexion and more mental alertness.

The Neck and Skull

As well as supporting the head, and being a passageway between the head and brain and the body, the neck allows head movements and is continuously stretched in a number of directions. Thanks to the neck, we can look up, down and rotate the head to look sideways or even almost behind us. The numerous muscles and joints of the face, neck and skull can greatly benefit from massage and bodywork.

The aims of massaging the skull area are to promote circulation and to induce relaxation. A tense scalp can slow down the superficial blood flow, hence aggravating hair loss and contributing to poor sleep and weak memory. By rubbing the scalp we can feel more alert and positive, reduce the pain of a headache and slow down or prevent hair loss.

Anatomy of the Neck

There are many important structures within the neck, making it a vital area. They are the spinal cord, the trachea (windpipe), the oesophagus as well as all the major blood vessels carrying blood to and from the head. The neck also contains the upper seven vertebrae of the spine and the thyroid and parathyroid glands. The neck is covered by a large muscle called the trapezius that originates from beneath the skull and reaches to the shoulders and down the thoracic spine. Consequently tension in the shoulder area or back, a very common occurrence, can also contribute to neck problems. Considering that the neck holds and moves the skull, it is a rather narrow and delicate structure which is prone to tense and painful muscles and stiff joints.

Many neck problems can, in various degrees, be helped by massage and bodywork. The strokes of massage, enhanced by essential oils, can stretch and relax sore and tense muscles. This relieves tension headaches and a feeling of stiffness that can often cause nausea, a feeling of being unwell and even mild depression. Articulatory techniques derived from either shiatsu or osteopathy can improve joint movement. This can either bring relief or prevent degenerative conditions like arthritis.

Cervical restrictions can affect the carotid and vertebral arteries which pass through the neck area as well as the nerve centre called the brachial plexus. This is why neck problems can

HEAD AND NECK MUSCLES

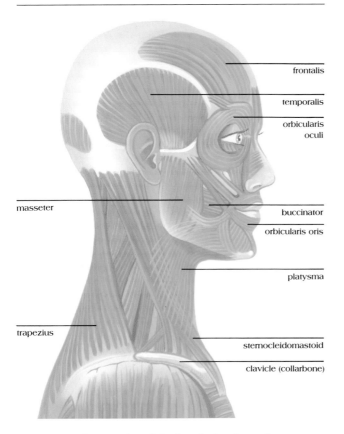

frontalis

temporalis

orbicularis oculi

masseter

buccinator

orbicularis oris

platysma

trapezius

sternocleidomastoid

clavicle (collarbone)

Massaging the muscles of the head stimulates the nerves and the flow of blood to the head and brain, and gives suppleness to the skin. This gives greater mental alertness and a feeling of well-being. Here are some of the muscles in a complicated system that controls head movement, biting, chewing and swallowing, and facial expression.

affect circulation. They can also cause sensations in the skin of the hands because the neck arteries are closely related to the arteries in the arm and various nerves descend all the way from the brachial plexus to the hands.

As an osteopath, I regularly see patients who are worried by symptoms in their hands, such as pins and needles or numbness. Often, after a few sessions working on both the neck and shoulders, their symptoms disappear.

Common Complaints

There are a number of common complaints for which massage and bodywork can be recom-

mended. According to the restrictions that you encounter, and the structures affected, you can choose the appropriate techniques. Longitudinal stretching techniques for the neck and head can alleviate uncomfortable muscle spasms, while articulations can help free the joints.

Neck arthritis

I have chosen the more common definition of this condition, although in medical books it is described under several names like cervical spondylosis and cervical osteoarthritis. (Cervical derives from the Latin, *cervix*, neck.) It is a classical case of wear and tear affecting the skeletal components of the neck.

Degenerative changes in the cervical spine can appear earlier than you might think, often in the thirties. One of the discs can be involved and the vertebrae might grow protuberances like spikes called osteophytes. The problem with the growth of ostephytes in the cervial vertebrae is that they can impinge on surrounding structures such as the nerves emanating from the neck joints. This causes severe pain and discomfort with reduced mobility. If the client is in severe pain, always recommend that they consult a doctor immediately and request an X-ray. X-rays can detect these changes and your doctor might prescribe medication and physiotherapy.

If the arthritis is not too advanced, gentle massage and manual traction can help alleviate this condition and contribute to preventing it from worsening. If the massage causes any pain, do not continue.

Non-specific neck pain

Many people complain of neck pain ranging in severity and from sporadic episodes to constant

---

ESSENTIAL OILS FOR THE NECK

For the massage, use a saucer containing 30 ml (2 tablespoons) of base oil, to which you can add two of drops of lavender oil and one drop of either chamomile, frankincense or geranium to relax the area and allay pain.

---

discomfort, yet no abnormal changes can be detected during routine medical investigations. The pain can start suddenly or build up over a period of time.

The pain is often due to excessive rotatory movements performed with the neck from an awkward angle during various forms of physical work, including exercise, dancing or sitting at a desk working on a typewriter or computer. We should be very aware of how we hold ourselves and move our necks, particularly during working hours. Unnatural and twisted positions can soon create persistent and worrying non-specific neck pain.

The muscles become tense often creating a spasm; the ligaments are sore due to unnatural stretching; the joints become stiff or, using bodywork terminology, 'jammed'. The action of massage and bodywork can be very useful and effective here. It relaxes the muscles and helps restore mobility to jammed joints.

Wry neck (torticollis)

In this condition the head is twisted to one side with considerable pain in the neck. The condition is greatly exacerbated when the person tries to straighten the head, which may, temporarily, remain in a tilted position. Some forms of torticollis are beyond the scope of this book. The one that I am referring to here occurs when the person complains of having woken up with a twisted, stiff and painful neck. The muscles on the side of the neck will be very tender and visibly in spasm. Most people have experienced an episode of torticollis at some time. It often occurs first thing in the morning, after sleeping with the neck in an uncomfortable position, which causes a muscle spasm.

In this case a gentle massage with relaxing oils like lavender can gradually warm and release the muscles and restore full mobility to the neck. If the pain is too severe a visit to a physiotherapist or osteopath might be required.

Whiplash

Whiplash injuries are a common cause of persistent neck pain. The injury occurs when one

---

> ### ESSENTIAL OILS FOR WHIPLASH INJURIES AND NECK PAIN
>
> Use a calming essential oil combination like two drops of lavender and one of frankincense to a saucer of 30 ml (2 tablespoons) of base oil. Another possible combination is one drop of lavender, one of chamomile and one of cypress. Gentle massage can encourage a fresh flow of blood to the area, hastening tissue repair and removing spasms and pain, thus making the person feel more comfortable.

---

vehicle strikes or is struck by another one; in the sudden and powerful collision, the person's head is rapidly thrown back or over-extended. This violent impact on a delicate area like the neck can cause extensive and persistent injury. If there are fractures, they must be fully healed before any form of massage or bodywork can be attempted directly on the area. If no fractures are present, a course of massage treatment, preferably under medical supervision, can help a whiplash injury.

In a whiplash injury most osteopaths believe that, although the neck is the main structure affected, all the rest of the spine is also affected particularly the lower back and sacrum. Therefore bodywork treatments on the back can also hasten the recovery of the neck area.

Hair loss

We should remember that, besides hormonal and hereditary causes, hair loss or brittleness can be due to factors like poor diet, stress and poor circulation. The latter is itself often due to lack of exercise.

We can massage the skull with or without some base oil, both ways are effective. If your scalp is dry and itchy some massage oil is recommended. Apply it a few hours before shampooing. To a saucer of 30 ml (2 tablespoons) of base oil you can add a drop of essential oil of rosemary which is a very good circulatory and toning herb. Rosemary should be avoided last thing at night, as it might keep you awake. Also avoid it if you suffer from migraines and high

---

NOURISHING YOUR HAIR

To nourish the roots of the hair mix together 50 g (2 oz) of nettle leaves (*Salvia sclarea*) and 25 g (1 oz) of sage (*Urtica dioica*). Prior to washing hair, make a cup of tea by infusing for ten minutes 5 mg (1 teaspoon) of the mixture to a cup of hot water. After shampooing, massage scalp by dipping your finger tips in the herbal tea.

---

blood pressure; use a drop of lavender instead. If you do not wish to apply oil you can, after shampooing, add a drop of your chosen essential oil to a jug of water and pour it over your wet hair while massaging the scalp.

Headaches and migraines

The word 'headache' covers any form of pain in the head. This sometimes can be the manifestation of a serious illness for which prompt medical attention is required. However, in the majority of cases the cause is not a serious pathological condition, and the advice given in this section could change for the better the lives of many headache and migraine sufferers.

Many forms of headache and migraine present a picture of symptoms that include muscular tension, particularly in the upper body; constriction of the neck vertebrae; poor digestion (*see Chapter Five, page 90*); and a state of general mental and emotional tension which is often accompanied by insomnia (*see Chapter Nine, page 140*). In the case of migraine there is an addition of the abnormal dilation and contraction of the circulatory vessels of the head causing severe pain. However, if the headache is caused by sinus congestion, refer to this chapter (*see page 130, step 5*), for ways of clearing mucus from the respiratory system.

In this chapter, through self-help massage, essential oils and herbs, you will be able to keep your neck and shoulders more flexible and free of tension. This will encourage better circulation to the head and help many forms of tension headache and migraine.

These time-tested techniques will also soothe and calm the skull nerves giving a clear head, better sleep and a more relaxed attitude. Headaches can also affect the face, so massage here too can be beneficial.

For tension headaches with possible constriction of blood vessels, the aim of the treatment is to encourage the patient to relax thus encouraging circulatory balance. Massage plays a vital role in achieving this result, but the hands-on approach can be further enhanced by various other natural and safe methods.

It makes sense to first assess your life style, including diet, and remove possible causative factors as far as possible. This can mean cutting down on too many stimulants such as coffee and alcohol as well as sugar and fatty foods, or even choosing a less stressful life style. It is important to learn how to relax: by releasing muscular tension, by inducing calm and regular breathing and by using calming visualizations (*see The Preparation, page 23*). Possible allergic triggers should be removed from the diet; many headache sufferers can pinpoint the ingestion of certain food prior to an attack.

ESSENTIAL OILS FOR HEADACHES AND MIGRAINES

Some essential oils diluted in a base oil can help to relieve headaches and tension. You can add two drops of any of the following essential oils or one drop each of two different oils to a saucer of 30 ml (2 tablespoons) of base oil: lavender, chamomile, neroli, orange peel, lemon balm and marjoram. These aromatic oils should be massaged particularly over the neck and shoulder areas. Lavender is considered one of the best relaxing and analgesic (pain removing) essential oils. However, because of its marked sedative properties it should not be used for more than two weeks consecutively. After that there should be a break of at least ten days before starting another course of applications. Chamomile and orange peel can also be used when digestive problems accompany the headache; for this condition also massage over the abdomen (*see page 93*). Neroli is particularly indicated for tension headaches with insomnia. Marjoram is useful when there is a respiratory complaint like sinusitis as well as the headache.

Massage for the Neck and Skull

The following bodywork and self-help techniques for the neck are a very effective way to improve its health and flexibility. The articulations maintain the natural movements of the neck, while the massage strokes keep the shoulder and neck muscles elastic and pain free. Nevertheless, always perform the following techniques very gently and slowly, and remember to carefully monitor the facial expressions of, or tension in, the receiver, in order to not stretch the neck beyond its capacity. If the neck is restricted, with time and patience you can deliver results. As the muscular spasms subside and the joints become freer, you will be able to stretch and free the delicate and vital neck area in stages without any need to force the pace. Massaging the skull, too, is both immensely pleasurable and stimulating.

1 *Kneeling above your partner's head, hold the neck in your hands covering the whole length of it with your palms. Visualize an Indian dancer side-shifting the neck from one side to the other. Gently side-shift the neck from one side to the other with your hands. Then repeat this technique three times. Remember to keep your shoulders relaxed, elbows well aligned.*

2 *Hold the neck as above. Gently side-bend the neck to one side. Repeat on the other side. Repeat twice on each side. If one side does not side-bend properly, hold it gently in a side-bend position and massage the opposite side to stretch and relax the muscles there.*

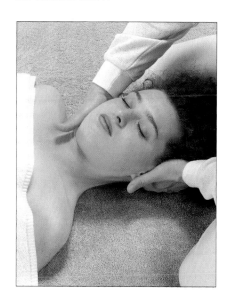

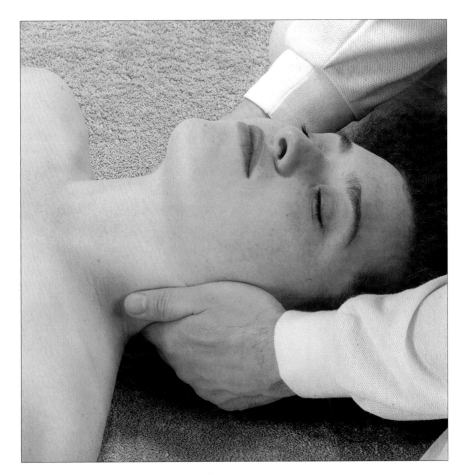

3 *Hold the neck with your hands slightly cupped and push up from the back of the neck with your index fingers, raising the chin as far as it will comfortably reach, which extends the neck. This movement originates from the middle part of the neck. Repeat three times. Can also be used on the upper and lower parts of the neck.*

4 *Cup one side of the neck with the length of your palm and support the side of the head with your other hand. This time slowly rotate the head to one side. Change your hand position and rotate the head, and then slowly to the other side. Repeat whole movement twice.*

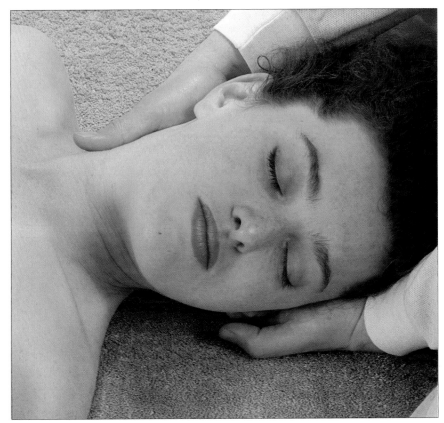

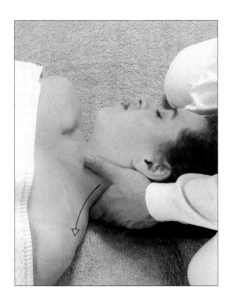

5 With the right hand place the tips of your fingers beneath the base of the skull and with your palms cradle the right side of the face and skull. Let the receiver relax their head and rest it in your right hand. Slightly pull the head away from the left shoulder. With the left hand gently stroke down the left side of the neck stretching its muscles (see left); rub the neck between the thumb and index finger. Repeat on opposite side.

6 Repeat same movement as above but this time rub with the three middle fingers (see right). Keep the head turned to one side.

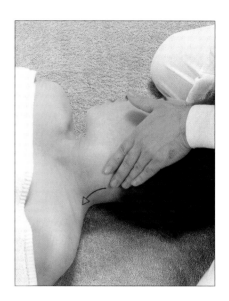

7 Hold the neck in the same way as in steps 5 and 6. This time gently squeeze the neck muscles up and down with your thumb and index finger. Let the squeezing movement be firm enough to pinch the flesh, but at the same time keep your fingers very relaxed. At no stage should this technique create a sense of discomfort in the receiver.

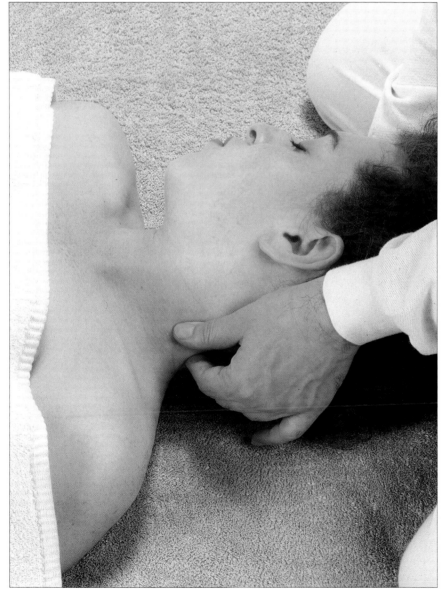

8 *With the head rotated to the right, place the tips of your fingers beneath the base of the skull and with your palms cradle the face and skull. Let the receiver relax the head on your hand. Gently pull the head and neck away from the left shoulder stretching the muscles of the shoulder and side of the neck. While the right hand pulls the head towards the right, with the left hand push the left shoulder downwards towards the left. Repeat for the other side. This forms a powerful stretch.*

9 *Place your palms beneath the base of the skull with the tips of the fingers reaching the lower part of the neck. Slowly raise the head and push the chin towards the chest. Stretch only as far as the neck can comfortably reach. As a variation, hold the base of the skull with one hand and massage the neck, stroking downward with gentle pressure with the other.*

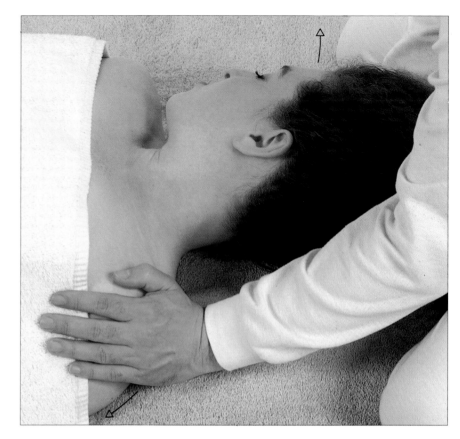

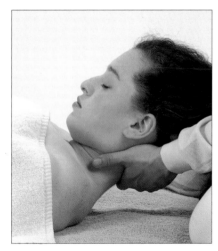

10 *Hold your hands beneath the neck, your index fingers folded in the lowest part of the neck and the fleshier part of the palms just beneath the base of the skull. Gently and slowly pull the neck towards you and stay in that position for a few seconds. Release the pull and repeat three times. Often performed in hospitals with a traction machine to release congestion between the cervical vertebrae.*

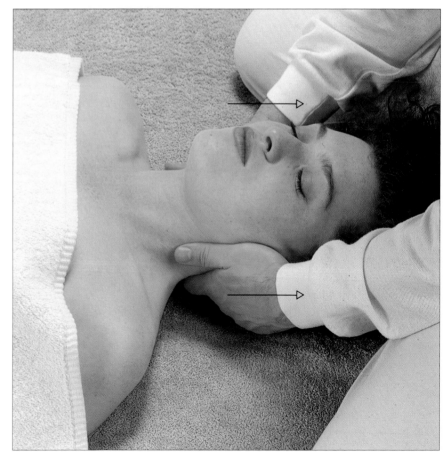

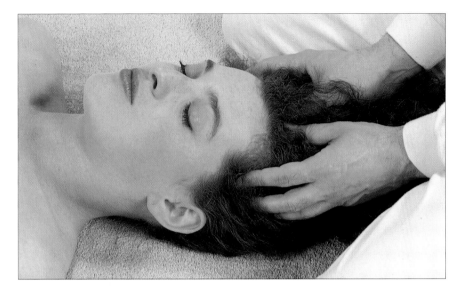

11 *Massage the scalp all over with your finger tips, as if you were shampooing the hair. This is a pleasurable technique that can greatly stimulate circulation in the scalp and head.*

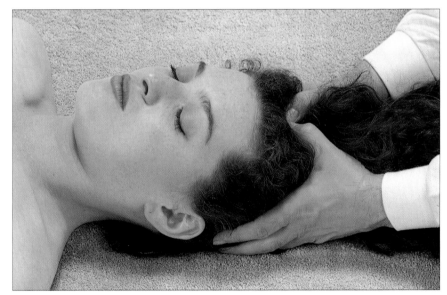

12 *With both thumbs press along the central line of the skull from the hairline to the top of the head. This technique stimulates the governing vessel meridian which stimulates the skull.*

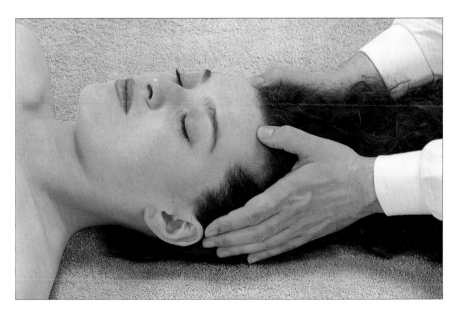

13 *Apply the same thumb pressure along the hairline with both thumbs starting at the middle of the forehead and then moving away from each other, all the way down the hairline as far as the ear.*

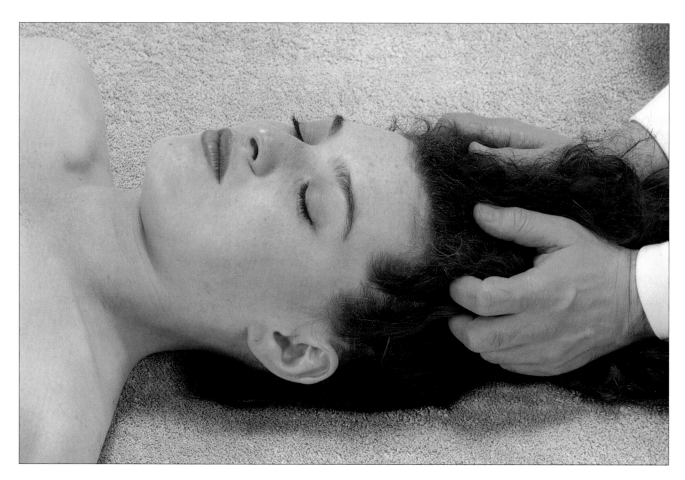

14 *Gently pull the hair in sections with the pull felt at scalp level. Do it slowly; the client should feel a pleasurable and relaxing sensation. Repeat a few times, changing the position of your hands each time, covering the whole skull.*

15 *Repeat the same technique as in step 11, this time with the receiver on their stomach, so the back of the head can be massaged. If you do not want to move the receiver, you can include this technique while massaging the back (see Chapter One, page 34).*

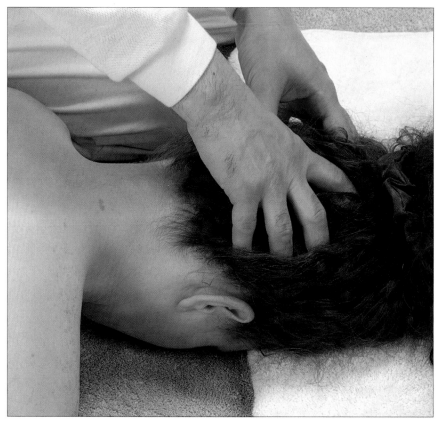

Self-help for the Neck and Skull

The emphasis of these self-help exercises is on performing slowing and carefully. The neck is a thin and flexible structure and therefore quite delicate and prone to injuries. In the past, some types of exercise have had to be modified to reduce the risk of neck injuries which were occurring. Such movements were at times too rapid, jerky and involved a succession of full neck rotations. This can over-stretch the ligaments and weaken the neck.

By performing slow half-rotations and gentle movements of side-bending, extension and flexion, you will be able to keep your neck flexible and possibly free of restrictions. Due to poor posture, strained movements and age, necks tend to become tense; many of the natural movements of the neck become restricted and painful. I have seen many people with very poor neck mobility who have spent years complaining of pain whenever they try to rotate their heads. They may also complain of other problems like tension headaches, and referred pain. In these cases insomnia is not uncommon because many sleeping positions in bed aggravate the neck. Massage, and especially self-help care, can work wonders for these common problems. The neck can be freed, for peaceful sleep and a pain-free life.

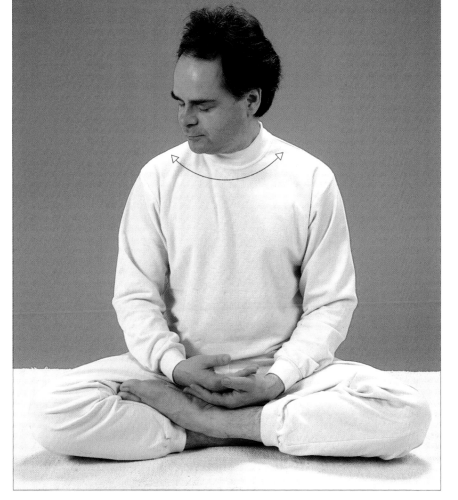

1 *Although this movement favours rotation of the neck, you should only half rotate the neck slowly looking from one shoulder to the other as far as you can go. Perform it slowly and gently, avoiding over-stretching the neck. Feel the muscles stretching gently.*

2 *Grab the opposite shoulder with one hand and squeeze its muscles with a rhythmic and continuous movement from the neck to the beginning of the arm and back for thirty seconds or so. Repeat with the other shoulder.*

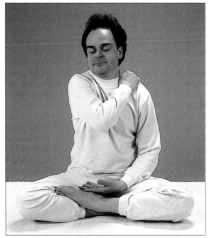

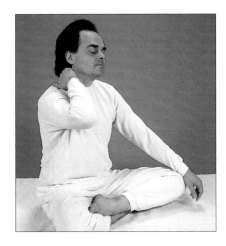

3 *Place the right hand on the right side of the neck and slightly pull the neck away from you to further expose the muscles. Rub and squeeze the neck up and down for thirty seconds. Repeat on the opposite side with the other hand.*

4 *Clasp both hands behind your neck with the fingers slightly interlocked (see right). Then slowly pull the hands away from each other towards the front of the body, rubbing the neck with the palms and fingers in the process. Repeat at least five times. This avoids tension accumulating in the neck and shoulder areas.*

5 *With very loose and relaxed fists gently percuss the skull all over. This technique should give a pleasant sensation and should never be painful. Do not do this if you have a headache or are experiencing a migraine attack.*

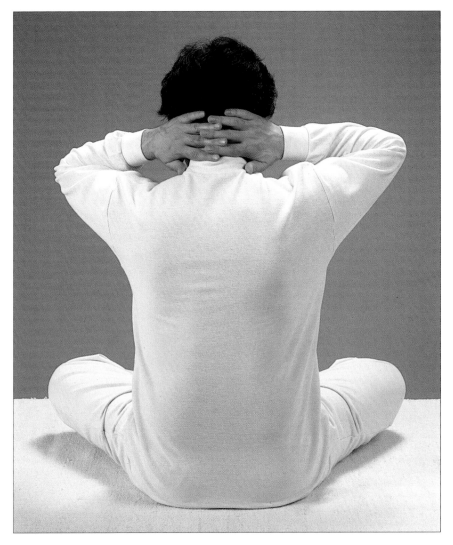

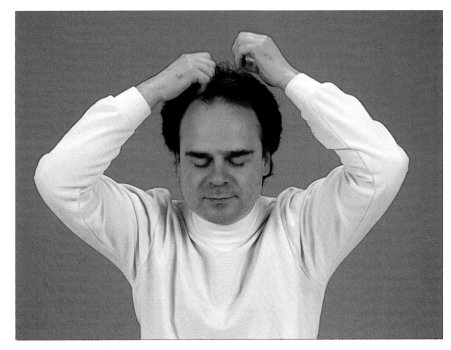

6 *Massage all over the scalp with the tips of your fingers, as if you were shampooing it. Always to be sure to massage in this fashion over the entire scalp, even if there are bald areas, for every part of the scalp will benefit from massage.*

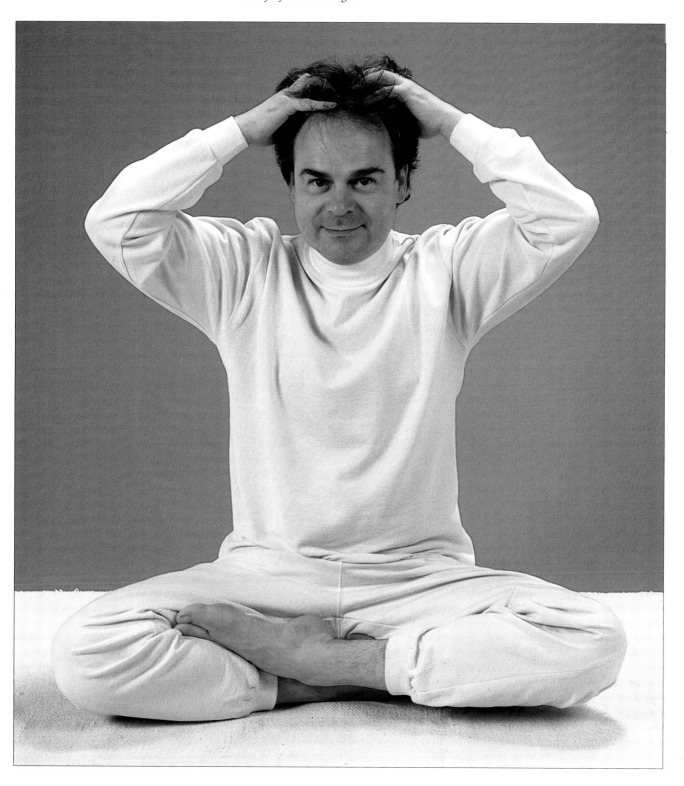

The Face

Sometimes we think that we can hide any complaints that we may carry within our bodies or minds. However, sooner or later they will show on our faces. The face and the eyes do not lie. We all want to feel good and to look good. The following advice will help improve your skin and the general appearance of your face. The best advice of all is to smile a lot and from the heart.

Healthy Skin, Youthful Face

No matter what your age, your face can always emanate a sense of youth and freshness. To achieve this it is important to think and feel with enthusiasm and have faith in life. Wallowing in negative emotions like resentment and anger can crease the face and create a look in the eyes that most people will find threatening. The condition of the facial skin reflects our general health, life style and diet. The latter should include lots of fresh fruit and vegetables, wholegrains and fibre. Chinese medicine believes that some of the main meridians flow through the face, mainly those of the colon, stomach and gall bladder. These are all digestive meridians. This is one of the reasons why too much junk food in the diet can have an adverse effect on the face.

Another extremely important step towards having a fresh and youthful face is massage, either administered by someone else or self-massage. These techniques, with the help of some essential oils and herbal preparations, will rejuvenate your face and maintain it as such. This process can be further enhanced with the help of exercises that will stretch and tone all the major muscles of the face (*see page 114*). This increases circulation to the face giving it a shining glow; by stimulating the secretion of moisture, it will soothe dry skin; it tones the skin, removing some of the wrinkles and avoiding future ones; and will also remove dead cells and encourage the growth of new ones, thereby keeping the face young-looking.

Practise this routine diligently every day, if possible, or at least once a week. Within a few weeks you will see gratifying results.

I like to add a word of caution about essential oils. The facial skin is very sensitive and occasionally some people can be allergic to one of the essential oils or ointments; therefore always apply them on a small patch and wait for a day to see if a reaction occurs.

In all the ointments I suggest the use of aqueous cream because it is made mainly from water and therefore very light and not greasy. If the skin is dry, you can use an emollient or moisturizing cream like vitamin E or borage.

Common Complaints

As we examine some of the most common problems of the facial skin, we can see how massage, accompanied by nutrition, essential oils and herbs can help. This is why some of the advice given includes blood-cleansing procedures because, as we have already mentioned, the health of the face reflects our general health, as well as the state of the blood.

Acne

This form of skin inflammation is especially prevalent among teenagers, when there is a change in the sebum secretion. The cause is uncertain, but is probably linked to increased levels of certain hormones. The moisture-producing sebaceous glands become over-active and they secrete too much sebum (grease). This grease blocks the hair follicles and sebaceous glands in the skin. Consequently pimples, lumps and blackheads are formed.

During an acute episode of inflammation it is best to massage the face very gently and, for

HERBAL TEA FOR ACNE

This herbal tea can be very useful in cleansing the blood and clearing the skin. It can be used to help most skin conditions. Mix together 25 g (1 oz) of dried burdock (*Arctium lappa*), heartsease (*Viola tricolor*), dandelion herb (*Taraxacum officinale*) and pellitory of the wall (*Parietaria officinalis*). In 600 ml (1 pint) of hot water, simmer for fifteen minutes 15 mg (1 tablespoon) of the mixture. Strain it and drink half a glass at least one hour before or after meals every few hours during a period of twenty-four hours.

If you can buy herbal tinctures, mix 50 ml (1¾ fl oz) each of the following herbs: burdock root (*Arctium lappa*), yellow dock root (*Rumex crispus*), dandelion root or leaves and heartsease. Pour 5 mg (1 teaspoon) of the mixture in a glass of water and drink twice a day at least one hour before or after meals.

ACUPRESSURE POINTS

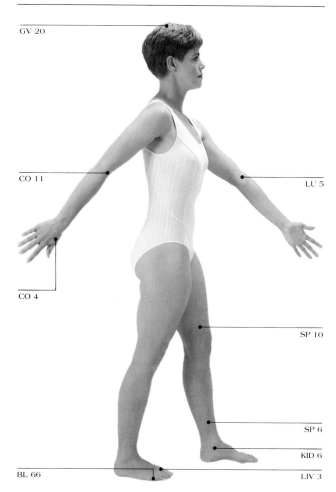

Acupressure points for the head and face can both soothe and revitalize. BL 66 helps relieve a sore or stiff neck. KID 6 and SP 6 help moisturize dry skin; LU 5 helps to dry oily skin. GV 20 lifts depression, eases headaches, migraine and dizziness and aids poor memory. SP 10, CO 4, CO 11 and LIV 3 all benefit the face in a variety of ways, reflected in a healthy, glowing skin.

only a few minutes, gradually increasing the length of this facial treatment as the condition slowly improves.

You can wash the face adding one drop of one of these essential oils in a bowl of water: lavender, rose, geranium, jasmine and sandalwood. After this application dry the face and massage it for a few minutes. Use only enough base oil to slightly moisten your fingers.

The following acupressure points contribute to revitalizing and cleansing the blood, benefitting a variety of skin conditions. Massage for a few minutes at least three times a week: SP 10 (*see Chapter Two, page 55*); CO 4, CO 11 and LIV 3 (*see Chapter Three, page 72*).

Dry skin

The skin has its own moisturizing secretion, the sebum, for protection against environmental factors like excessive heat, cold and pollution. If the glands are under-active, the skin will be dry and flaky and with age will tend to wrinkle prematurely. Massage, enhanced with essential oils, aims to increase circulation to the face and to stimulate the sebaceous glands.

In warm countries the skin can become too dry because of the heat; in cold countries the skin can also become very dry because of the

CREAM FOR DRY SKIN

The following ointment applied last thing at night can also help dry skin. Use as a base 30 g (1 oz) of aqueous cream and 30 g (1 oz) of a moisturizing cream like avocado, vitamin E or borage. Add 15 ml (1 tablespoon) each of the tincture of chickweed (*Stellaria media*) and marsh mallow root (*Althaea officinalis*); two drops each of the essential oils of rose and of geranium. Mix very well.

effects of central heating; it is advisable to place humidifiers over the radiators. If you spend a lot of time in a polluted atmosphere, use a protective cream in the morning. Also, wash your face adding to the water one drop of any of the following essential oils: rose, geranium or jasmine.

The following acupressure points are useful for dry skin: KID 6 and SP 6. Rub them both three times a week for a couple of minutes. Both these points increase the Yin energy in the body and, as we have already seen, the Yin pole regulates coolness and moisture in the body.

Oily skin

In this condition the sebaceous glands that secrete sebum to moisturize and protect the skin are overactive causing a greasy appearance. Again massage and essential oils can be helpful in regulating this problem. Also, avoid deep-fried food, such as fish and deep-fried potatoes, and high fat content food like full fat cheese.

CREAM FOR OILY SKIN

The following ointment applied last thing at night can also help in controlling an oily skin. In 60 g (2¼ oz) of aqueous cream add 15 ml (1 tablespoon) each of tincture of plantain (*Plantago officinalis*) and of marigold (*Calendula officinalis*), two drops each of lavender and sandalwood. Mix very well.

You can wash your face adding one drop of any of the following essential oils: lavender, bergamot or sandalwood.

The following acupressure points are beneficial for oily skin: CO 4 (*see Chapter Three, page 72*) and LU 5 (*see Chapter Four, page 83*). Rub each one gently for a couple of minutes three times a week.

Acupressure Points for the Head

The following points can promote well being in the region of the head.

Governing Vessel 20 (GV 20). Draw an imaginary line between the upper tips of the two ears. This point lies in the middle of the skull at the point where the two lines meet. GV 20 has an harmonizing effect on the nervous system and brain. It lifts depression while calming and relaxing the mind. It can also be used for headaches and migraines, dizziness and poor memory.

BL 66 can help soothe a sore or stiff neck (*see Chapter One, page 33*). Dry skin can be helped with SP 6 (*see Chapter Two, page 55*) and KID 6 (*see Chapter Seven, page 108*). SP 10 (*see Chapter Two, page 55*), CO 4, CO 11 and LIV 3 (*see Chapter Three, page 72*) are all beneficial to a variety of skin conditions. CO 4 (*see Chapter Three, page 72*) and LU 5 (*see Chapter Four, page 83*) help alleviate oily skin.

Massage for the Face

If you and your partner or friends practise these techniques on each other, you will increase the bond between you. You will soon realize that, not only does a caring touch bring people together and create unity, but also that each of you is making a positive contribution to the health, well-being and youthful looks of the other participants.

If you are a therapist, you will already know how grateful the recipients are to you for the sense of pleasant relaxation and glowing, healthy skin that you bring to them through face massage.

Some time ago, when I was practising in Rome, my clients included actors and actresses. They came to me before each show because they felt that massage and bodywork for the face and head improved their performances by relaxing the facial muscles which then became even more expressive.

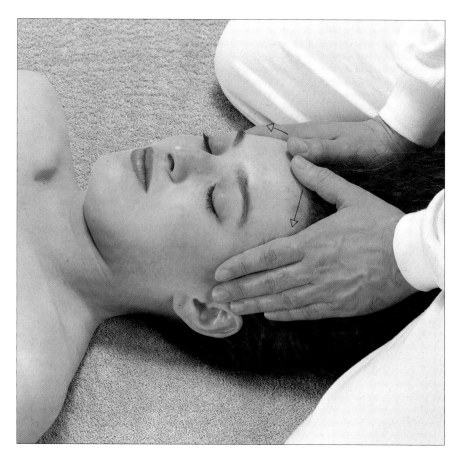

1 Place both thumbs in the middle of the upper part of the forehead just beneath the hairline (see left). Rub in a straight motion with the thumbs moving away from each other to the temples. Repeat in the middle part of the forehead and again in the lower part just above the eyebrows.

2 Repeat the same motion as above, but this time instead of the thumb use the three middle fingers. Keep the fingers close together throughout this stroke.

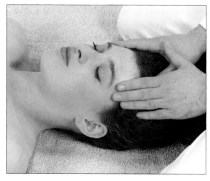

3 Place the middle three fingers over the temples and gently rub them in a circular motion towards the scalp for a couple of minutes. This technique has a very soothing and calming effect.

4 With thumbs and index fingers start pinching the eyebrows from the bridge of the nose to their far ends; you can work your way back to the bridge of the nose.

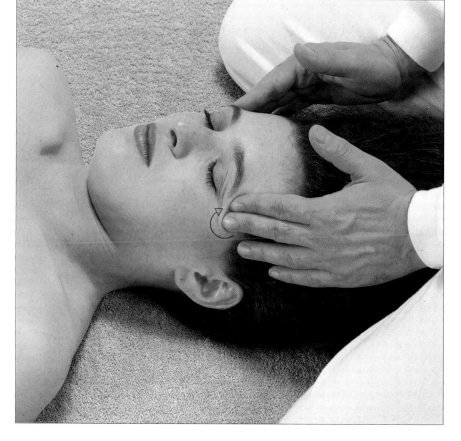

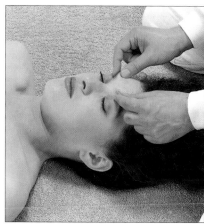

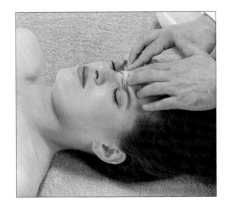

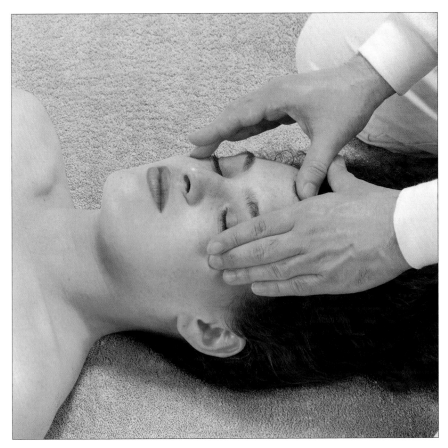

5 Place the middle fingers just above the end of the eyebrows and rub towards the nose (see above). *Repeat five or six times. This helps to clear congested sinuses.*

6 Place the middle fingers in the point where the eyes meet the bridge of the nose. *From there gently rub in a circular motion around the eye area passing just beneath the eyebrows and above the cheekbones. Do not rub directly above the eye socket; stay 2.5 cm (1 in) below it.*

7 Place the middle three fingers on each cheek and stroke firmly *towards the temples. Return and repeat three times. As you massage towards the temples, feel the skin being stretched gently.*

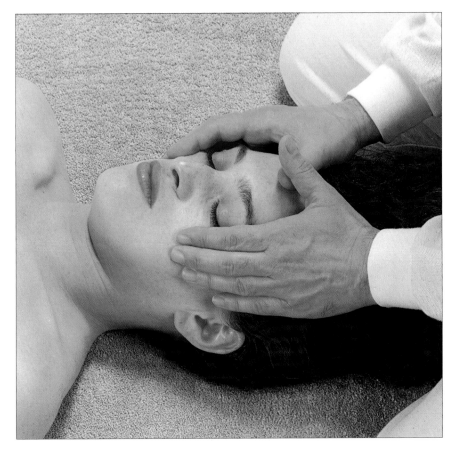

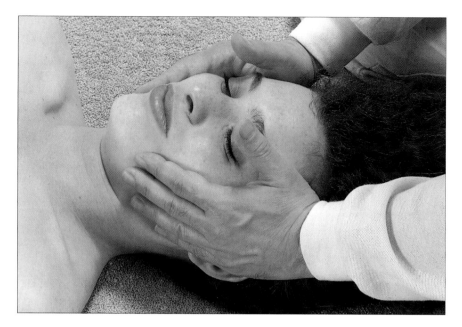

8 *Place the three middle fingers where the jaw meets the chin. Stroke all the way to the temples. Return and repeat three times.*

9 *With thumbs and index fingers, starting from the middle of the chin pinch along all the length of the jaw (see below). This technique can release the tension that is often stored in this area.*

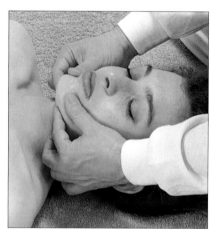

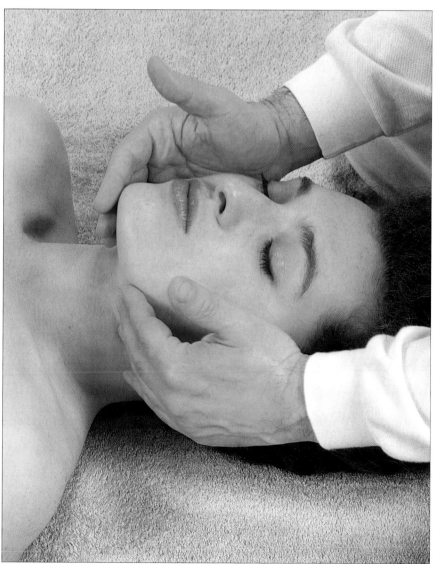

10 *This stroke is excellent to reduce double chins. Position both hands just below the chin and stroke with each hand alternately towards the base of the neck (see left). Keep the chin in an upright position to assist the downward stroke. Repeat five times.*

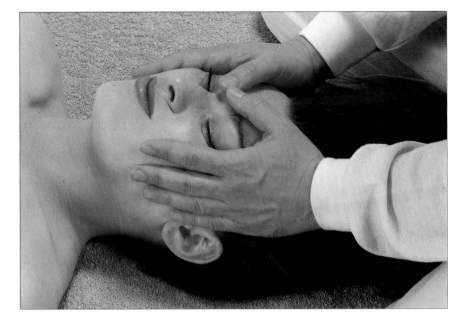

11 *Place both hands with open palms over the face, resting the thumbs between the eyebrows, and slowly rub all the way up to the temples. Return and repeat this technique three times.*

12 *Turn client onto their stomach and massage the back of the neck. Use your fingers to squeeze gently and pull through the length of the neck.*

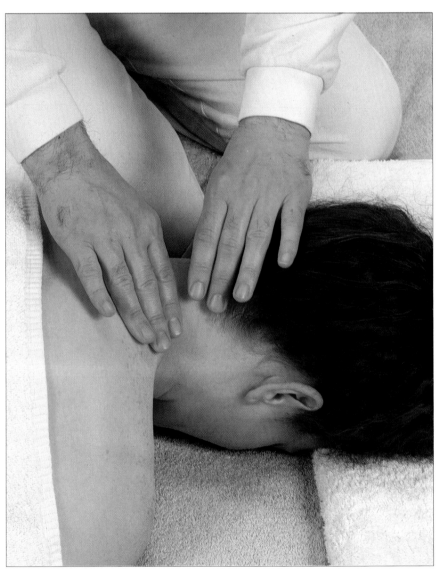

Self-help for the Face

This self-massage should be practised at least three times a week for five months for it to yield visible results. The pressure should be constant and strong enough to stimulate circulation, but not so heavy as to irritate the skin. If performed correctly, after the massage you should feel warmth and a glow on your face. Within a few weeks there should be a clear improvement in the condition of your skin. Alternate carrying out the technique between morning and night. If you find it difficult to stick to a regular routine, do not worry.

The advantage of these self-help techniques is that they can be performed at almost any time, in an office, while travelling, even when relaxing and watching television.

These self-massage techniques will remove dead cells and bring in a new supply of blood to the face and head. This in turn encourages the elimination of toxins and promotes cellular regeneration. At the same time the exercises will strengthen the muscles of the face, helping to avoid tissue sagging prematurely and encourages a firm, healthy facial skin.

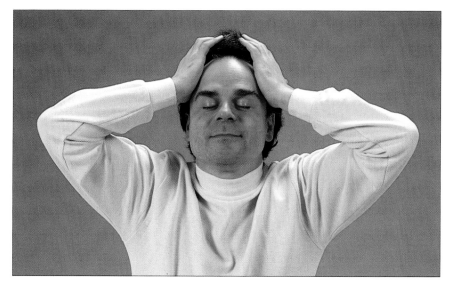

1 *Place the heels of both hands in the middle of the upper part of the forehead. Rub with both palms moving away from each other till you reach the temples. Repeat this technique in the middle part of the forehead and in the lower area just above the eyebrows.*

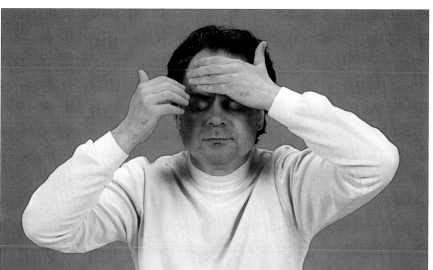

2 *Place one hand over the forehead. With the hand in contact with the skin, stroke the forehead through its entire length from one temple to the other. Next change hands rapidly and stroke in the same way in the opposite direction. Repeat this alternate stroke three times.*

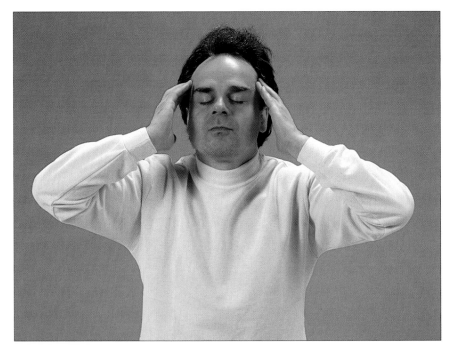

3 *Place your three middle fingers on your temples and rub them in a slow circular motion in the direction of the scalp.*

4 *With thumbs and index fingers start pinching the eyebrows from the bridge of the nose to their ends; you can work your way back again from there to the bridge of the nose. Repeat several times.*

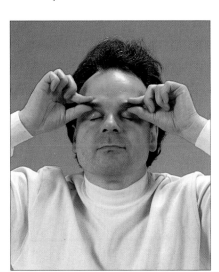

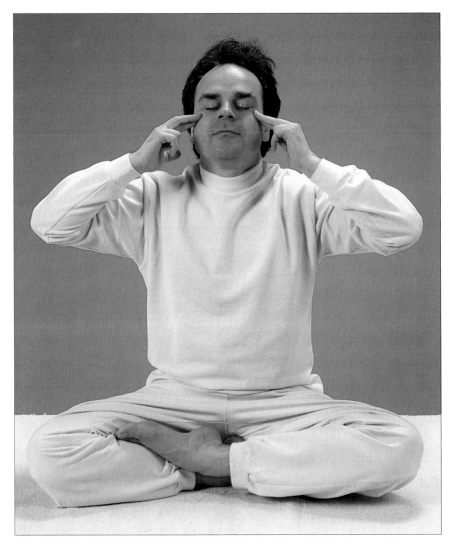

5 *Place the middle fingers in the point where the eye meets the bridge of the nose. From there gently rub in a circular motion around the eye area passing just beneath the eyebrows and above the cheekbones. Do not rub directly above the eye socket, never beneath it. Stay 2.5 cm (1 in) away from the eye socket.*

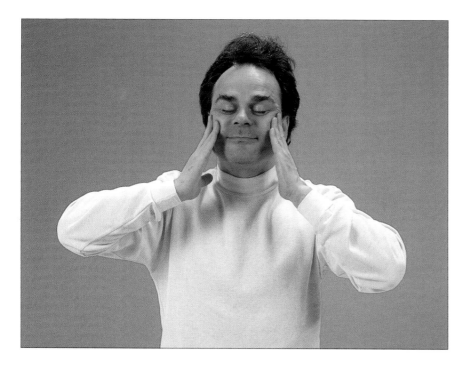

6 *Place the middle three fingers on each cheek, just below the cheek bones, and stroke towards the temples. Repeat three times.*

7 *With thumbs, middle and index fingers pinch all along the length of the jaw (see below). Repeat this technique three times. This is an excellent technique for releasing tension.*

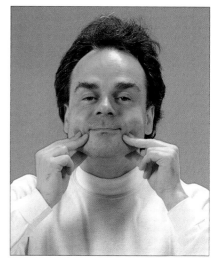

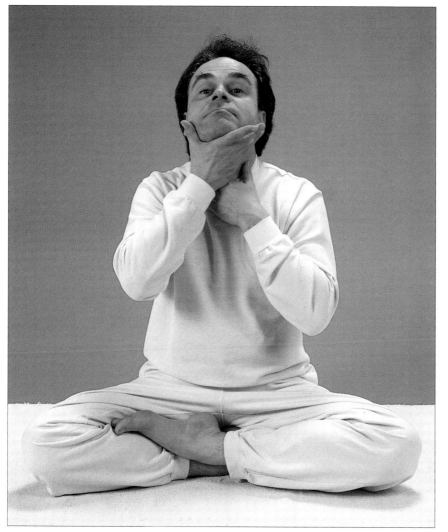

8 *Position one hand on top of the other just below the chin and stroke with each hand alternately towards the base of the neck. Always keep the chin in an upright position to assist the downward stroke. Repeat this technique five times. This stroke is excellent to help reduce double chins and smoothe the skin of the neck.*

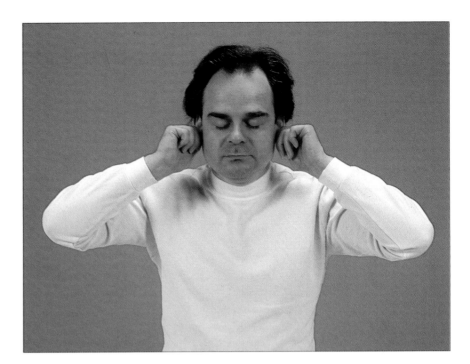

9 *With the thumbs and index fingers grab hold of the ears and gently pull them stroking them in the process. Repeat all along the length of the ears.*

10 *Place both hands with open palms over the face and then slowly rub all the way up to the temples. Return and repeat slowly three times.*

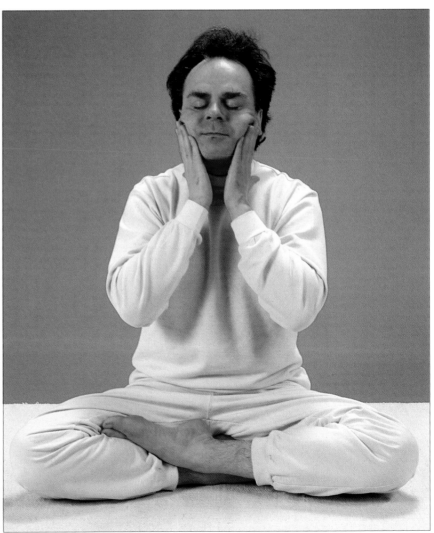

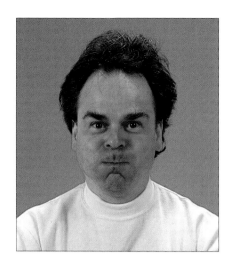

11 *Pull a face by trying to blow out while keeping the mouth firmly closed (see left). This technique helps to strengthen many muscles of the face.*

12 *Lift your chin up as far as possible and pull a face, always remembering to particularly stretch the muscles beneath your chin (see right). This exercise firms the muscles under the chin, and is good for reducing double chins. This is a very useful technique because you can do it almost anywhere.*

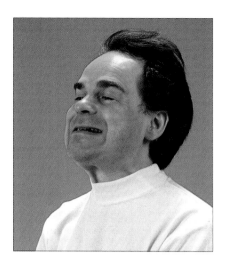

13 *This yoga exercise (see left), called the lion pose, stretches and stimulates almost every muscle of the face as well as releasing pent up anger and frustration! Kneel with your wrists resting on your knees; then open your mouth and jaw stretching all your face as wide as possible and roar like a lion imagining that you are one! Do this exercise for thirty seconds.*

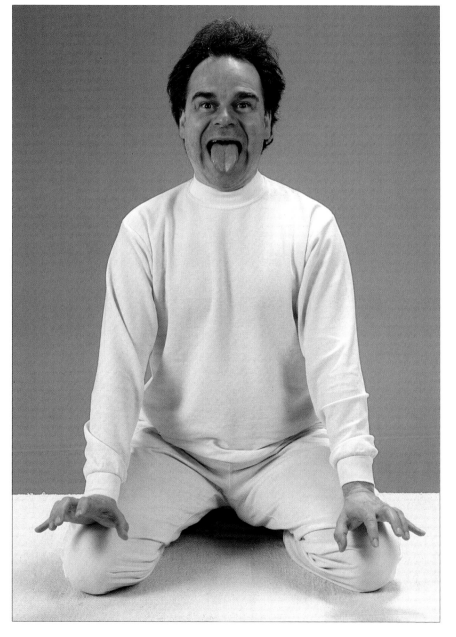

CHAPTER NINE

Happy and Relaxed

The skills of massage can be learned by anyone, the benefits enjoyed by everyone. A health-giving and caring touch proves its worth in every session. At the end of a massage a tense and debilitated person will feel invigorated and, at the same time, soothed.

Renewed Vitality and Optimism

As well as improving general health, massage can have a profound effect on our emotional and mental well being. Powerful and painful emotions affect our conscious and subconscious minds. They can also disturb the functioning of the nervous system by either tensing or collapsing our musculature. They can contract the nerves that control breathing and digestion, causing nervous asthma, various digestive disorders, and ulcerations.

Sadness and depression, along with its resulting lethargy, can weaken our muscles, curve our spine and sink our chest; some believe this can lead to weak immunity.

Massage and bodywork increase circulation with many related benefits. It imparts warmth and a glow to our bodies and minds; relaxes tense and contracted muscles, making us feel calm and more conciliatory; it awakens and tones weak and lax muscles, giving us renewed vitality and optimism.

The techniques in this chapter are intended to infuse the receiver with a deep sense of relaxation, to release pent-up emotions, and above all to instil a sense of trust and nurturing. They have been included because they are the best way to bring a massage session to an end, leaving the recipient peaceful and grateful for a new sense of cheerfulness and tranquillity.

In reality all the massage techniques in this book, if performed when appropriate, can help rejuvenate and revitalize the nervous system. Nerves are present in every part of the body and each individual may store emotions in different areas and in different ways: one recipient may lock their emotions in the abdomen, while another may hold them in the chest or back; some receivers feel very relaxed when their feet are massaged, others their head and so on.

The following advice in part makes use of the emotional understanding of Chinese medicine; work with it and see if and when it can be of help. Over many centuries millions of people have found this approach to be beneficial.

Common Complaints

From time to time most of us suffer from complaints like insomnia or depression that can diminish our enjoyment of life. Often these problems can be greatly improved through the loving and comforting touch of massage.

Depression

No one can claim that massage is a cure for depression. However, a soothing and caring touch can alleviate the hopelessness and sense

---

ESSENTIAL OILS TO ALLEVIATE DEPRESSION

Refer to the Properties of Essential Oils *(see page 15)* to find the most suitable essential oil for the client's physical and emotional make up, from the following: jasmine, rose, orange peel, lemon balm, bergamot, rosemary or clary sage. Add three drops to a saucer of 30 ml (2 tablespoons) base oil. Use one oil or mix as many as three different ones (one drop of each).

---

of isolation that accompanies this state of mind. At the same time the invigorating effects of a full-body massage can help stimulate a little more enthusiasm and zest in the recipient.

For depression, Chinese medicine advocates the treatment of acupressure points along the heart and spleen meridian. With a circular motion massage the following points for two minutes three times a week: PE 6 and SP 6 (*see Chapter Two, page 55*); ST 36 (*see Chapter Five, page 92*); HE 3 (*see this chapter, page 140*).

Anger

This emotion can be an appropriate reaction to a form of abuse or injustice, but often it seems to be the result of unresolved past events when we once felt neglected and humiliated; we store this anger and it overflows at the slightest confrontation or misunderstanding.

In Chinese medicine anger is considered to be an emotion of the liver, therefore anger can be treated by rubbing LIV 3 (*see Chapter Three, page 72*) with a circular motion for three minutes two or three times a week. You can also gently massage the liver area of the abdomen. Massage around the upper body and feet relaxes a body tensed with stored anger.

Sadness and grief

Sadness is considered, in Chinese medicine, to be an emotion of the lungs. An image that always comes to my mind is that of the roman-tic poets and artists of the last two centuries, who in fact were often ill with serious pulmonary illnesses. These emotions can also be

---

DEFLECT SADNESS WITH ESSENTIAL OILS

Add 30 ml (2 tablespoons) of base oil to a saucer, then two drops each of the essential oils of marjoram and bergamot. If you know your massage partner well and the depth of the complaint, modify this combination; use any oils that you feel are more in tune with your massage partner by first referring to Properties of Essential Oils (*see page 15*).

ACUPRESSURE POINTS

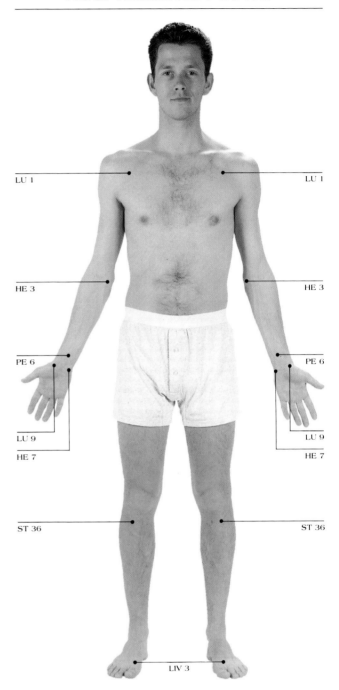

Acupressure points can help throw off powerful, negative emotions and conditions, such as anger, depression, sadness, and insomnia. However, some points, like HE 3, can positively encourage the more joyful and spiritual aspects of our nature. To ease sadness and depression, use PE 6, SP 6 (see page 55), ST 36, LU 1, LU 9 and HE 3. For anger use LIV 3. To help insomnia use the points PE 6, SP 6 and HE 7.

the result of our inability to cope with the loss of a loved one or even of valued possessions.

With a circular motion massage the following acupressure points for two minutes two or three times a week: LU 1 (*see Chapter Four, page 83*) and LU 9 (*see below*).

Insomnia

Most of us experience an occasional night when we cannot fall asleep. This may be due to causes such as worry, or even a late meal that sits uncomfortably in the stomach; but for many people insomnia can become chronic. Lack of sleep can greatly debilitate, and reduce mental alertness and concentration. Massage helps by soothing the nervous system and the mind. You can also practise self-massage to relax the neck and shoulders. Choose essential oils that are calming like chamomile, lavender and neroli.

Massage the following acupressure points in a circular motion for two minutes each before retiring: PE 6 and SP 6 (*see Chapter Two, page 55*) and HE 7 (*see Chapter Seven, page 108*). Many herbal combinations are available in health food shops and pharmacies that can promote sleep without the drowsiness associated with most drug-oriented sleeping tablets.

Always go to sleep with a light stomach and do not take stimulant drinks like coffee and tea at night. Also useful are the relaxation exercises given in The Preparation (*see page 23*).

Acupressure Points

The use of these points promotes a happy and relaxed frame of mind.

Heart 3 (HE 3). This point is at the very inside end of the elbow crease on the inside of the arm. Pressure on HE 3 strengthens the joyful aspects of the spiritual side of the heart. It lifts depression indicated by low spirits, grief, lack of enthusiasm and so on.

Lung 9 (LU 9). Follow the uppermost wrist crease, to find this point lying in its most external side just below the thumb. It strengthens the lungs, is good for chronic conditions of the respiratory system, but do not tone during an acute respiratory infection. It can help to lift sadness and gloominess.

The following points can be found as follows: PE 6 and SP 6 (*see Chapter Two, page 55*); CO 11 and LIV 3 (*see Chapter Three, page 72*); LU 1 (*see Chapter Four, page 83*); St 36 (*see Chapter Five, page 92*) and HE 7 (*see Chapter Seven, page 108*).

Finishing a Massage Sequence

It is very important to begin and end a massage on the right note. Also, do not chat too much during a session. Restlessness and boredom is communicated to the receiver, the comforting physical contact of massage is interrupted, then suddenly broken.

I always encourage my students to practise a few minutes of meditation to compose themselves prior to meeting the receiver. This enables them to concentrate and give a massage in an attentive frame of mind. Accompany a massage session with gentle music, if the receiver enjoys this. Total silence is best when the receiver needs to release pent-up emotions.

How we end a massage is equally important. The techniques here, because of their soothing and relaxing nature, form an appropriate sequence to end a massage session. The receiver must not be jarred by an abrupt transition from a state of relaxation and passivity to sudden activity. These techniques are intended to gradually ease the transition from the languid relaxation of massage back to a busy life style.

Monitor the breathing of your massage partner carefully while performing the following techniques. You might notice at first that it becomes more tense and erratic. Do not worry. Just remember to keep yourself relaxed.

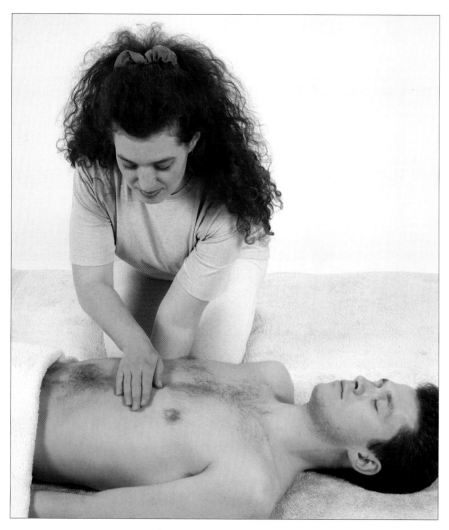

1 Kneeling beside your partner, place one hand on the tip of the sternum and the other hand on the corresponding area beneath the spine. Breathe deeply and relax your shoulders and arms. Keep this hold, communicating a sense of nurturing. After a few minutes you will feel them take a deep breath and calm their breathing, followed by a general relaxation of the whole body. If you do not achieve this at first, do not worry. It will happen eventually. Caution: *Do not hold this position for more than three minutes.*

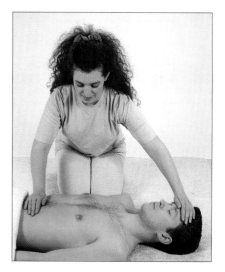

2 Remaining in the same position, place one hand on the abdomen and one on the forehead. Again relax and calm yourself and communicate a sense of tranquillity and nurturing. Hold this position for up to three minutes.

3 Kneel above the receiver's head and place their head on your lap. This is a comforting position. With your fingertips stroke over the forehead and head. Then comb through the hair, gently stroking the scalp (see left). If the receiver is bald simply stroke over the scalp.

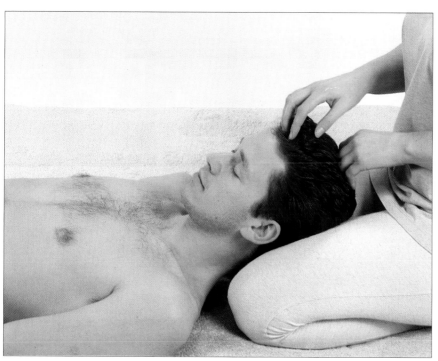

141

Index

Acknowledgements

I acknowledge the forefathers of osteopathy such as Still, Littlejohn and Fryette for the founding work they did in this field to whom I am indebted. In addition, I would like to thank all my teachers, students and patients, who over the last twenty-five years have enriched my life and often have become my best friends; my girl-friend Julia for all her patient and kind support; the staff at Eddison Sadd for their creative spirit and good humour; and Pat Pierce for editing the book through the Christmas holidays.

Let this book come alive! The author has produced a full two-hour video, based on *Massage and Bodywork for Health*, demonstrating massage and bodywork techniques, self-massage and self-help exercises, plus the location of acupressure points.

To order your copy, please write to: Expressions, PO Box 5513, London W8 5WE, United Kingdom; or telephone (415) 469 7774.

EDDISON · SADD EDITIONS

Art Director Elaine Partington

Art Editor Hilary Krag

Project Editor Zoë Hughes

Copy-editors Barbara Nash and Pat Pierce

Indexer Dorothy Frame

Production Hazel Kirkman and Charles James